ATS-132 ADMISSION TEST SERIES

This is your PASSBOOK for...

National Optometry Boards (NOB)

Test Preparation Study Guide
Questions & Answers

NLC®
NATIONAL LEARNING CORPORATION®

COPYRIGHT NOTICE

National Learning Corporation

212 Michael Drive, Syosset, NY 11791
(516) 921-8888 • www.passbooks.com
E-mail: info@passbooks.com

PASSBOOK® SERIES

THE *PASSBOOK® SERIES* has been created to prepare applicants and candidates for the ultimate academic battlefield – the examination room.

At some time in our lives, each and every one of us may be required to take an examination – for validation, matriculation, admission, qualification, registration, certification, or licensure.

Based on the assumption that every applicant or candidate has met the basic formal educational standards, has taken the required number of courses, and read the necessary texts, the *PASSBOOK® SERIES* furnishes the one special preparation which may assure passing with confidence, instead of failing with insecurity. Examination questions – together with answers – are furnished as the basic vehicle for study so that the mysteries of the examination and its compounding difficulties may be eliminated or diminished by a sure method.

This book is meant to help you pass your examination provided that you qualify and are serious in your objective.

The entire field is reviewed through the huge store of content information which is succinctly presented through a provocative and challenging approach – the question-and-answer method.

A climate of success is established by furnishing the correct answers at the end of each test.

You soon learn to recognize types of questions, forms of questions, and patterns of questioning. You may even begin to anticipate expected outcomes.

You perceive that many questions are repeated or adapted so that you can gain acute insights, which may enable you to score many sure points.

You learn how to confront new questions, or types of questions, and to attack them confidently and work out the correct answers.

You note objectives and emphases, and recognize pitfalls and dangers, so that you may make positive educational adjustments.

Moreover, you are kept fully informed in relation to new concepts, methods, practices, and directions in the field.

You discover that you are actually taking the examination all the time: you are preparing for the examination by "taking" an examination, not by reading extraneous and/or supererogatory textbooks.

In short, this PASSBOOK®, used directedly, should be an important factor in helping you to pass your test.

NATIONAL OPTOMETRY BOARDS (NOB)

EXAM DESCRIPTIONS

The National Optometry Board administers two types of examinations: complete, integrated comprehensive examination parts; and a short, limited-scope, special examination. The three parts of the standard "National Boards" are designed primarily for different stages of a candidate's optometric education and training. Special examinations, on the other hand, are designed primarily for practitioners who wish to broaden their scope of practice in accordance with expanding practice statutes. The National Board examinations include:

Part I (Basic Science)
Part II (Clinical Science)
Part III (Patient Care).

The three comprehensive examination Parts are designed as a complete set of examinations to assess the cognitive, psychomotor, affective, and communication skills that are essential for entry-level optometric practice. Parts I and II are approximately 1.5 days in length; Part III is 1.0 day in length.

Each examination Part is developed by a broad geographic cross-section of the optometric community, which includes faculty members, state board members, and practitioners. These subject-matter experts comprise test development committees that are responsible for developing a specific portion or section of an examination Part. For written examinations, this activity consists of reviewing, editing, and selecting test items written by the National Board's team of consultant item writers and case writers. All test items are scrutinized for accuracy, conformance to the specific test content outline, and appropriateness for entry-level difficulty.

Each examination development committee is represented on one of the three examination councils, each of which also has representation by a liaison member from the Board of Directors. Every council is responsible for the integration of the component sections of one of the Parts, and may be responsible for a related special examination (e.g., TMOD). Throughout this process, the examination councils are responsible for monitoring and maintaining the entry-level appropriateness of all test content.

Each examination council also directs and reviews the scoring of the corresponding examination Part. This process includes the identification of flawed test items that should be deleted from scoring and any irregularities that might exert either a random or systematic deleterious effect on the scoring. The councils are accountable to the Board of Directors, which is ultimately responsible for the validity of the examinations, and the reliability of the examination results.

Each of the three examination Parts of the National Board is administered twice each year. Part I (Basic Science) is administered in August and December; Part II (Clinical Science) is administered in April and December; and Part III (Patient Care) is administered in April and August. The Clinical Skills section for the April examination of Patient Care is administered over three weekends, in order to accommodate all candidates in the one-to-one (examiner-to-candidate) format.

Both administrations of the respective Parts are designed to be alike with respect to content, difficulty, and pass-fail cutoff scores. As these examinations are integrated tests, they each have one overall pass-fail standard that must be met. This allows candidates to compensate for areas of relative subject-matter weakness by other areas of relative strength. However, candidates who fail the overall Part must repeat the entire Part.

The Treatment and Management of Ocular Disease (TMOD) examination consists of 150 multiple-choice items. This examination assesses the cognitive skills deemed essential for utilizing pharmacologic agents for the therapeutic management of ocular disease and trauma, as defined by the broadest state practice statute.

Optometry students take the equivalent of this examination within the Part II (Clinical Science) examination. Therefore, the stand-alone TMOD examination is targeted primarily for practitioners who wish to expand their scope of practice. Students are eligible to sit for the stand-alone TMOD examination during April of their fourth academic year. However, as noted earlier, optometry students typically meet the TMOD requirement within the Part II (Clinical Science) examination. Students who pass Part II (Clinical Science) at the December administration of their fourth academic year, but fail the embedded TMOD section, may sit for the stand-alone TMOD examination at the following April administration. The stand-alone TMOD examination is administered in one 3-3/4 hour session during April and August.

EXAM CONTENT

PART I: Basic Science

- Human Biology
- Ocular/Visual Biology
- Theoretical, Ophthalmic & Physiological Optics
- Psychology

PART II: Clinical Science

- Systemic Conditions
- Ocular Disease/Trauma
- Refractive/Oculomotor/Sensory Integrative Conditions
- Perceptual Conditions
- Public Health
- Legal and Ethical Issues

PART III: Patient Care

- Clinical Skills
- Patient Assessment and Management (PAM)

SAMPLE TEST ITEMS

The National Board uses multiple-choice test items in its assessment of cognitive skill. Multiple-choice items are preferred because their ability to sample material from the universe of optometric knowledge promotes test validity. In addition, multiple-choice items are objective, allow high speed and efficient scoring, and enhance the sophistication of statistical analysis that yields high levels of test reliability and detailed score reporting.

Many multiple-choice tests that candidates have taken prior to the National Board required systematic familiarization with the specific and perhaps unique formats that were used. This type of preparation is not necessary for successful or even optimal performance on the National Board examinations because there are no contrived formats that are used. While National Board test items will often test complex optometric material and require higher level cognitive processes (e.g., problem-solving skills) in order to correctly answer the item, the specific item format is simple and direct.

Each test item consists of a stem that contains the question part of the item, and usually four or five options, one of which is the correct or best response. Occasionally, an item will have as few as three options if three options represent the universe of possible answers (e.g., the effect of a drug on intraocular pressure can either be to increase, decrease, or not change it). Most National Board test items contain four options.

Some items will contain pictorial or other graphic material such as a fundus photo, an anatomical schematic, or a data table or graph. The item may then require the visual material to be interpreted in order for the correct answer to be selected. National Board test items do not include potentially confusing combination response options such as "none of the above," "all of the above," or subsets such as "a and b above." Thus, candidates who have taken multiple-choice examinations should not need any special preparation for the National Board format. Therefore, preparation for the multiple-choice examinations can concentrate entirely on optometric content rather than on familiarization with test format.

The stem of many National Board items contains a superlative (e.g., MOST), a pejorative (e.g., LEAST), or a negative (e.g., NOT). Many test items on the examination will contain items written with one of these adjectives or adverbs. The purpose of this type of item is not to mislead, "trick," or "split hairs," but rather, to represent some of the types of clinical decisions that practitioners often confront. For example, a patient may be treated with several regimens; however, the selection criterion is typically the MOST effective treatment with the LEAST likely discomfort. In other items, any one of several treatments may be equally effective, but there is one that should NOT be prescribed. Therefore, when confronting a test item of this nature, candidates should respond to the item as they would to the corresponding actual clinical situation. To try to prevent any misreading of the test item, the superlative, pejorative, and negative descriptors are capitalized and underlined.

Some test items refer to patients or subjects with non-normal conditions. Unless the test item provides information suggestive of an underlying non-normal condition, candidates should assume that the referenced patient is normal.

HOW TO TAKE A TEST

You have studied long, hard and conscientiously.

With your official admission card in hand, and your heart pounding, you have been admitted to the examination room.

You note that there are several hundred other applicants in the examination room waiting to take the same test.

They all appear to be equally well prepared.

You know that nothing but your best effort will suffice. The "moment of truth" is at hand: you now have to demonstrate objectively, in writing, your knowledge of content and your understanding of subject matter.

You are fighting the most important battle of your life—to pass and/or score high on an examination which will determine your career and provide the economic basis for your livelihood.

What extra, special things should you know and should you do in taking the examination?

I. YOU MUST PASS AN EXAMINATION

A. WHAT EVERY CANDIDATE SHOULD KNOW

Examination applicants often ask us for help in preparing for the written test. What can I study in advance? What kinds of questions will be asked? How will the test be given? How will the papers be graded?

B. HOW ARE EXAMS DEVELOPED?

Examinations are carefully written by trained technicians who are specialists in the field known as "psychological measurement," in consultation with recognized authorities in the field of work that the test will cover. These experts recommend the subject matter areas or skills to be tested; only those knowledges or skills important to your success on the job are included. The most reliable books and source materials available are used as references. Together, the experts and technicians judge the difficulty level of the questions.

Test technicians know how to phrase questions so that the problem is clearly stated. Their ethics do not permit "trick" or "catch" questions. Questions may have been tried out on sample groups, or subjected to statistical analysis, to determine their usefulness.

Written tests are often used in combination with performance tests, ratings of training and experience, and oral interviews. All of these measures combine to form the best-known means of finding the right person for the right job.

II. HOW TO PASS THE WRITTEN TEST

A. BASIC STEPS

1) Study the announcement

How, then, can you know what subjects to study? Our best answer is: "Learn as much as possible about the class of positions for which you've applied." The exam will test the knowledge, skills and abilities needed to do the work.

Your most valuable source of information about the position you want is the official exam announcement. This announcement lists the training and experience qualifications. Check these standards and apply only if you come reasonably close to meeting them. Many jurisdictions preview the written test in the exam announcement by including a section called "Knowledge and Abilities Required," "Scope of the Examination," or some similar heading. Here you will find out specifically what fields will be tested.

2) Choose appropriate study materials

If the position for which you are applying is technical or advanced, you will read more advanced, specialized material. If you are already familiar with the basic principles of your field, elementary textbooks would waste your time. Concentrate on advanced textbooks and technical periodicals. Think through the concepts and review difficult problems in your field.

These are all general sources. You can get more ideas on your own initiative, following these leads. For example, training manuals and publications of the government agency which employs workers in your field can be useful, particularly for technical and professional positions. A letter or visit to the government department involved may result in more specific study suggestions, and certainly will provide you with a more definite idea of the exact nature of the position you are seeking.

3) Study this book!

III. KINDS OF TESTS

Tests are used for purposes other than measuring knowledge and ability to perform specified duties. For some positions, it is equally important to test ability to make adjustments to new situations or to profit from training. In others, basic mental abilities not dependent on information are essential. Questions which test these things may not appear as pertinent to the duties of the position as those which test for knowledge and information. Yet they are often highly important parts of a fair examination. For very general questions, it is almost impossible to help you direct your study efforts. What we can do is to point out some of the more common of these general abilities needed in public service positions and describe some typical questions.

1) General information

Broad, general information has been found useful for predicting job success in some kinds of work. This is tested in a variety of ways, from vocabulary lists to questions about current events. Basic background in some field of work, such as sociology or economics, may be sampled in a group of questions. Often these are principles which have become familiar to most persons through exposure rather than through formal training. It is difficult to advise you how to study for these questions; being alert to the world around you is our best suggestion.

2) Verbal ability

An example of an ability needed in many positions is verbal or language ability. Verbal ability is, in brief, the ability to use and understand words. Vocabulary and grammar tests are typical measures of this ability. Reading comprehension or paragraph interpretation questions are common in many kinds of civil service tests. You are given a paragraph of written material and asked to find its central meaning.

IV. KINDS OF QUESTIONS

1. Multiple-choice Questions

Most popular of the short-answer questions is the "multiple choice" or "best answer" question. It can be used, for example, to test for factual knowledge, ability to solve problems or judgment in meeting situations found at work.

A multiple-choice question is normally one of three types:

- It can begin with an incomplete statement followed by several possible endings. You are to find the one ending which best completes the statement, although some of the others may not be entirely wrong.
- It can also be a complete statement in the form of a question which is answered by choosing one of the statements listed.
- It can be in the form of a problem – again you select the best answer.

Here is an example of a multiple-choice question with a discussion which should give you some clues as to the method for choosing the right answer:

When an employee has a complaint about his assignment, the action which will best help him overcome his difficulty is to

A. discuss his difficulty with his coworkers
B. take the problem to the head of the organization
C. take the problem to the person who gave him the assignment
D. say nothing to anyone about his complaint

In answering this question, you should study each of the choices to find which is best. Consider choice "A" – Certainly an employee may discuss his complaint with fellow employees, but no change or improvement can result, and the complaint remains unresolved. Choice "B" is a poor choice since the head of the organization probably does not know what assignment you have been given, and taking your problem to him is known as "going over the head" of the supervisor. The supervisor, or person who made the assignment, is the person who can clarify it or correct any injustice. Choice "C" is, therefore, correct. To say nothing, as in choice "D," is unwise. Supervisors have and interest in knowing the problems employees are facing, and the employee is seeking a solution to his problem.

2. True/False

3. Matching Questions

Matching an answer from a column of choices within another column.

V. RECORDING YOUR ANSWERS

Computer terminals are used more and more today for many different kinds of exams.

For an examination with very few applicants, you may be told to record your answers in the test booklet itself. Separate answer sheets are much more common. If this separate answer sheet is to be scored by machine – and this is often the case – it is highly important that you mark your answers correctly in order to get credit.

VI. BEFORE THE TEST

YOUR PHYSICAL CONDITION IS IMPORTANT

If you are not well, you can't do your best work on tests. If you are half asleep, you can't do your best either. Here are some tips:

1) Get about the same amount of sleep you usually get. Don't stay up all night before the test, either partying or worrying—DON'T DO IT!
2) If you wear glasses, be sure to wear them when you go to take the test. This goes for hearing aids, too.
3) If you have any physical problems that may keep you from doing your best, be sure to tell the person giving the test. If you are sick or in poor health, you relay cannot do your best on any test. You can always come back and take the test some other time.

Common sense will help you find procedures to follow to get ready for an examination. Too many of us, however, overlook these sensible measures. Indeed, nervousness and fatigue have been found to be the most serious reasons why applicants fail to do their best on civil service tests. Here is a list of reminders:

- Begin your preparation early – Don't wait until the last minute to go scurrying around for books and materials or to find out what the position is all about.
- Prepare continuously – An hour a night for a week is better than an all-night cram session. This has been definitely established. What is more, a night a week for a month will return better dividends than crowding your study into a shorter period of time.
- Locate the place of the exam – You have been sent a notice telling you when and where to report for the examination. If the location is in a different town or otherwise unfamiliar to you, it would be well to inquire the best route and learn something about the building.
- Relax the night before the test – Allow your mind to rest. Do not study at all that night. Plan some mild recreation or diversion; then go to bed early and get a good night's sleep.
- Get up early enough to make a leisurely trip to the place for the test – This way unforeseen events, traffic snarls, unfamiliar buildings, etc. will not upset you.
- Dress comfortably – A written test is not a fashion show. You will be known by number and not by name, so wear something comfortable.
- Leave excess paraphernalia at home – Shopping bags and odd bundles will get in your way. You need bring only the items mentioned in the official notice you received; usually everything you need is provided. Do not bring reference books to the exam. They will only confuse those last minutes and be taken away from you when in the test room.

- Arrive somewhat ahead of time – If because of transportation schedules you must get there very early, bring a newspaper or magazine to take your mind off yourself while waiting.
- Locate the examination room – When you have found the proper room, you will be directed to the seat or part of the room where you will sit. Sometimes you are given a sheet of instructions to read while you are waiting. Do not fill out any forms until you are told to do so; just read them and be prepared.
- Relax and prepare to listen to the instructions
- If you have any physical problem that may keep you from doing your best, be sure to tell the test administrator. If you are sick or in poor health, you really cannot do your best on the exam. You can come back and take the test some other time.

VII. AT THE TEST

The day of the test is here and you have the test booklet in your hand. The temptation to get going is very strong. Caution! There is more to success than knowing the right answers. You must know how to identify your papers and understand variations in the type of short-answer question used in this particular examination. Follow these suggestions for maximum results from your efforts:

1) Cooperate with the monitor

The test administrator has a duty to create a situation in which you can be as much at ease as possible. He will give instructions, tell you when to begin, check to see that you are marking your answer sheet correctly, and so on. He is not there to guard you, although he will see that your competitors do not take unfair advantage. He wants to help you do your best.

2) Listen to all instructions

Don't jump the gun! Wait until you understand all directions. In most civil service tests you get more time than you need to answer the questions. So don't be in a hurry. Read each word of instructions until you clearly understand the meaning. Study the examples, listen to all announcements and follow directions. Ask questions if you do not understand what to do.

3) Identify your papers

Civil service exams are usually identified by number only. You will be assigned a number; you must not put your name on your test papers. Be sure to copy your number correctly. Since more than one exam may be given, copy your exact examination title.

4) Plan your time

Unless you are told that a test is a "speed" or "rate of work" test, speed itself is usually not important. Time enough to answer all the questions will be provided, but this does not mean that you have all day. An overall time limit has been set. Divide the total time (in minutes) by the number of questions to determine the approximate time you have for each question.

5) Do not linger over difficult questions

If you come across a difficult question, mark it with a paper clip (useful to have along) and come back to it when you have been through the booklet. One caution if you do this – be sure to skip a number on your answer sheet as well. Check often to be sure that you have not lost your place and that you are marking in the row numbered the same as the question you are answering.

6) Read the questions

Be sure you know what the question asks! Many capable people are unsuccessful because they failed to read the questions correctly.

7) Answer all questions

Unless you have been instructed that a penalty will be deducted for incorrect answers, it is better to guess than to omit a question.

8) Speed tests

It is often better NOT to guess on speed tests. It has been found that on timed tests people are tempted to spend the last few seconds before time is called in marking answers at random – without even reading them – in the hope of picking up a few extra points. To discourage this practice, the instructions may warn you that your score will be "corrected" for guessing. That is, a penalty will be applied. The incorrect answers will be deducted from the correct ones, or some other penalty formula will be used.

9) Review your answers

If you finish before time is called, go back to the questions you guessed or omitted to give them further thought. Review other answers if you have time.

10) Return your test materials

If you are ready to leave before others have finished or time is called, take ALL your materials to the monitor and leave quietly. Never take any test material with you. The monitor can discover whose papers are not complete, and taking a test booklet may be grounds for disqualification.

VIII. EXAMINATION TECHNIQUES

1) Read the general instructions carefully. These are usually printed on the first page of the exam booklet. As a rule, these instructions refer to the timing of the examination; the fact that you should not start work until the signal and must stop work at a signal, etc. If there are any special instructions, such as a choice of questions to be answered, make sure that you note this instruction carefully.

2) When you are ready to start work on the examination, that is as soon as the signal has been given, read the instructions to each question booklet, underline any key words or phrases, such as least, best, outline, describe and the like. In this way you will tend to answer as requested rather than discover on reviewing your paper that you listed without describing, that you selected the worst choice rather than the best choice, etc.

3) If the examination is of the objective or multiple-choice type – that is, each question will also give a series of possible answers: A, B, C or D, and you are called upon to select the best answer and write the letter next to that answer on your answer paper – it is advisable to start answering each question in turn. There may be anywhere from 50 to 100 such questions in the three or four hours allotted and you can see how much time would be taken if you read through all the questions before beginning to answer any. Furthermore, if you

come across a question or group of questions which you know would be difficult to answer, it would undoubtedly affect your handling of all the other questions.

4) If the examination is of the essay type and contains but a few questions, it is a moot point as to whether you should read all the questions before starting to answer any one. Of course, if you are given a choice – say five out of seven and the like – then it is essential to read all the questions so you can eliminate the two that are most difficult. If, however, you are asked to answer all the questions, there may be danger in trying to answer the easiest one first because you may find that you will spend too much time on it. The best technique is to answer the first question, then proceed to the second, etc.

5) Time your answers. Before the exam begins, write down the time it started, then add the time allowed for the examination and write down the time it must be completed, then divide the time available somewhat as follows:
    - If 3-1/2 hours are allowed, that would be 210 minutes. If you have 80 objective-type questions, that would be an average of 2-1/2 minutes per question. Allow yourself no more than 2 minutes per question, or a total of 160 minutes, which will permit about 50 minutes to review.
    - If for the time allotment of 210 minutes there are 7 essay questions to answer, that would average about 30 minutes a question. Give yourself only 25 minutes per question so that you have about 35 minutes to review.

6) The most important instruction is to read each question and make sure you know what is wanted. The second most important instruction is to time yourself properly so that you answer every question. The third most important instruction is to answer every question. Guess if you have to but include something for each question. Remember that you will receive no credit for a blank and will probably receive some credit if you write something in answer to an essay question. If you guess a letter – say "B" for a multiple-choice question – you may have guessed right. If you leave a blank as an answer to a multiple-choice question, the examiners may respect your feelings but it will not add a point to your score. Some exams may penalize you for wrong answers, so in such cases only, you may not want to guess unless you have some basis for your answer.

7) Suggestions
    a. Objective-type questions
        1. Examine the question booklet for proper sequence of pages and questions
        2. Read all instructions carefully
        3. Skip any question which seems too difficult; return to it after all other questions have been answered
        4. Apportion your time properly; do not spend too much time on any single question or group of questions
        5. Note and underline key words – all, most, fewest, least, best, worst, same, opposite, etc.
        6. Pay particular attention to negatives
        7. Note unusual option, e.g., unduly long, short, complex, different or similar in content to the body of the question
        8. Observe the use of "hedging" words – probably, may, most likely, etc.

9. Make sure that your answer is put next to the same number as the question
10. Do not second-guess unless you have good reason to believe the second answer is definitely more correct
11. Cross out original answer if you decide another answer is more accurate; do not erase until you are ready to hand your paper in
12. Answer all questions; guess unless instructed otherwise
13. Leave time for review

b. Essay questions
   1. Read each question carefully
   2. Determine exactly what is wanted. Underline key words or phrases.
   3. Decide on outline or paragraph answer
   4. Include many different points and elements unless asked to develop any one or two points or elements
   5. Show impartiality by giving pros and cons unless directed to select one side only
   6. Make and write down any assumptions you find necessary to answer the questions
   7. Watch your English, grammar, punctuation and choice of words
   8. Time your answers; don't crowd material

8) Answering the essay question

Most essay questions can be answered by framing the specific response around several key words or ideas. Here are a few such key words or ideas:

M's: manpower, materials, methods, money, management
P's: purpose, program, policy, plan, procedure, practice, problems, pitfalls, personnel, public relations

a. Six basic steps in handling problems:
   1. Preliminary plan and background development
   2. Collect information, data and facts
   3. Analyze and interpret information, data and facts
   4. Analyze and develop solutions as well as make recommendations
   5. Prepare report and sell recommendations
   6. Install recommendations and follow up effectiveness

b. Pitfalls to avoid
   1. Taking things for granted – A statement of the situation does not necessarily imply that each of the elements is necessarily true; for example, a complaint may be invalid and biased so that all that can be taken for granted is that a complaint has been registered
   2. Considering only one side of a situation – Wherever possible, indicate several alternatives and then point out the reasons you selected the best one
   3. Failing to indicate follow up – Whenever your answer indicates action on your part, make certain that you will take proper follow-up action to see how successful your recommendations, procedures or actions turn out to be
   4. Taking too long in answering any single question – Remember to time your answers properly

EXAMINATION SECTION

EXAMINATION SECTION
TEST 1

DIRECTIONS: Each question or incomplete statement is followed by several suggested answers or completions. Select the one that BEST answers the question or completes the statement. *PRINT THE LETTER OF THE CORRECT ANSWER IN THE SPACE AT THE RIGHT.*

1. After it is produced, aqueous humor flows through the ______ to fill the anterior chamber of the eye. 1.____

   A. pupil
   B. canal of Schlemm
   C. trabecular mesh
   D. Cloquet's canal

2. The inferior ophthalmic vein 2.____

   A. has more tributaries than the superior ophthalmic vein
   B. runs below the inferior rectus and enters the cavernous sinus
   C. passes through the optic canal
   D. communicates with the pterygoid plexus

3. The "duplicity theory" of vision refers to the existence of two 3.____

   A. areas in the brain to where visual input is conducted
   B. hard-wired pathways from each eye to the visual system
   C. competing theories about how light is processed into neural input
   D. different kinds of sensory input, photopic and scotopic

4. Of the following, the vitreous humor is MOST adherent to the 4.____

   A. ora serrata
   B. fovea
   C. ciliary body
   D. asteroid hyaloses

5. If a monocular image is located at a particular point in one eye, fusion is possible as long as the other monocular image is positioned within a small region around the corresponding point in the other eye. This area is known as ______ area. 5.____

   A. Nyquist's
   B. Panum's
   C. Muller's
   D. Purkinje's

6. Receptor potentials of the photoreceptors, and the electrical responses of most of the other natural elements in the retina, are unique in that they are local, graded potentials. The exception is the ______ cells, which transmit all-or-none potentials over appreciable distances. 6.____

A. ganglion
B. bipolar
C. amacrine
D. horizontal

7. Which of the following is NOT a result of the normal aging process of the cornea? 7.____

A. Decreased density in endothelium
B. Increased thickness of corneal stroma
C. Decreased translucency
D. Increased thickness of Bowman's membrane

8. The "rod-free" portion of the retina, where visual acuity is greatest, is the 8.____

A. fovea centralis
B. macula lutea
C. dura
D. optic disk

9. Which of the following types of crystallin is found mostly in the nucleus of the lens? 9.____

A. alpha-
B. beta-
C. gamma-
D. delta

10. The ophthalmic nerve 10.____

A. is both a motor and a sensory nerve
B. receives sympathetic fibers from the internal carotid plexus
C. branches three times after entering the orbit
D. lies above the trochlear nerve in the cavernous sinus

11. Which of the following does NOT affect visual acuity? 11.____

A. illumination
B. length of visual stimulus
C. red-green color blindness
D. pupil size

12. Optic disk drusen is NOT typically associated with 12.____

A. angioid streaks
B. venous obstruction
C. age-related macular degeneration
D. visual field abnormalities

13. The lipid layer of the tear film is formed by the _______ glands. 13.____

A. Meibomian
B. Wolfring
C. Müller
D. Krause

14. The first branch of the ophthalmic artery is the ______ artery. 14.____

A. palpebral
B. ciliary
C. supratrochlear
D. central retinal

15. Which of the following is NOT required for rhodopsin regeneration? 15.____

A. Ascorbic acid
B. Separation of all trans-retinal from the opsin
C. Retinal isomerase
D. Darkness

16. In most people, optic nerve myelinization terminates at 16.____

A. the uvea
B. the optic papilla
C. Gunn's dots
D. the lamina cribrosa

17. Which of the following cranial nerves carries parasympathetic outflow from the brain stem? 17.____

A. Oculomotor
B. Optic
C. Trigeminal
D. Glossopharyngeal

18. Ocular hypertension induced by steroids 18.____

A. is not commonly associated with dexamethasone
B. is reversible without regard to the duration of use
C. rarely occurs if the steroid is used for less than a year
D. depends on the potency of the steroid used

19. The trochlear nerve 19.____

A. innervates the ipsilateral superior oblique muscle
B. has a nucleus located in the cerebral aqueduct in the midbrain
C. is a pure motor nerve
D. enters the orbit through the annulus of Zinn

20. As the human eye develops, the 20.____

A. choroid becomes the first structure in the body to produce melanin
B. macular development is completed after birth
C. optic cup begins to close posteriorly
D. macular development begins in the third month of gestation

21. Which of the following is NOT a direct-acting cholinergic agonist? 21.____

A. carbachol
B. pilocarpine
C. echothiophate iodide
D. atropine

22. Which of the following drugs increases the risk of retinal detachment? 22.____

A. Latanoprost
B. Brimonidine
C. Atropine
D. Echothiophate

23. Actions of the superior oblique muscle include 23.____

A. intorsion
B. extorsion
C. elevation
D. adduction

24. Which of the following processes is NOT involved in the "near triad?" 24.____

A. Accommodation
B. Miosis
C. Adduction
D. Convergence

25. The optic chiasm's blood supply does NOT come by way of the ______ artery. 25.____

A. ophthalmic
B. anterior communicating
C. posterior communicating
D. anterior cerebral

26. When light is directed into one pupil, the pupil of the other eye constricts along with it. This is known as the ______ light reflex. 26.____

A. Argyll Robertson
B. consensual
C. afferent
D. efferent

27. Which of the following does NOT occur when light strikes the rhodop-sin of the eye? 27.____

A. Rods decrease their neurotransmitter release
B. Rhodopsin is bleached
C. Rhodopsin binds to retinal molecules
D. Sodium ion channels are closed

28. Visual information processing in the retina involve the formation of three images. The third image is formed in the ______ cells. 28.____

A. ganglion
B. Müller
C. horizontal
D. amacrine

29. The geniculocalcarine fibers from the lateral half of the lateral geniculate body terminate on the 29.____

A. lateral half of the lateral geniculate body
B. medial half of the lateral geniculate body
C. superior lip of the calcarine fissure
D. inferior lip of the calcarine fissure

30. The seventh layer of the retina is known as the 30.____

A. Inner plexiform
B. Outer plexiform
C. Outer nuclear
D. Inner nuclear

31. In the ______, the suprachiasmatic nuclei form connections that synchronize endocrine and other circadian rhythms with the light-dark cycle. 31.____

A. optic chiasm
B. amygdala
C. pineal gland
D. hypothalamus

32. If damaged, the ciliary ganglion will cause 32.____

A. mydriasis of the contralateral eye
B. mydriasis of the ipsilateral eye
C. ptosis of the contralateral eyelid
D. ptosis of the ipsilateral eye

33. Which of the following results in the effect of blue colors appearing brighter at dusk? 33.____

A. Pulfrich's phenomenon
B. Aubert's phenomenon
C. Lowe's syndrome
D. Purkinje's shift

34. The individual frames of a motion picture are perceived as one continuous movement because the frames are presented at a rate above the 34.____

A. color contrast threshold
B. pursuit threshold
C. critical fusion frequency
D. visual threshold

35. The ora serrata 35.____

A. adheres loosely to the vitreous
B. lies interior to the junction of the choroid and the ciliary body
C. composes a part of the pars plana
D. forms a regular margin around the pars optica

36. The X, or small ganglion, cells of the retina 36.____

A. are concerned with movement
B. combine responses from different kinds of cones
C. are concerned with color vision
D. are concerned with stereopsis

37. ______ nystagmus is a consequence of head rotation. 37.____

A. Vestibular
B. Optokinetic
C. Caloric
D. Pendular

38. The retina and pigment epithelium originate from embryonic neural tissue that continues forward as a bilayered epithelium to cover the ciliary body and the 38.____

A. zonule fibers
B. posterior surface of the lens
C. posterior surface of the iris
D. anterior surface of the lens

39. Which of the following nerves is NOT a branch of the ophthalmic nerve? 39.____

A. Frontal
B. Lacrimal
C. Nasociliary
D. Zygomatic

40. The detection of movement is mediated by the ______ cells of the retina, which conduct information to the geniculate body. 40.____

A. X, or small ganglion, cells
B. Y, or large ganglion, cells
C. bipolar
D. amacrine

41. Which of the following structures is embryologically derived from the mesoderm? 41.____

A. Eyelashes
B. Lacrimal gland
C. Sclera
D. Conjunctival epithelium

42. Damage to Meyer's loop causes a(n) 42.____

A. bitemporal hemianopia
B. homonymous hemianopia with macular sparing
C. blindness in the contralateral eye
D. superior quadrantopia

43. The constriction of the pupil is mediated by nerve fibers in the 43.____

A. ciliary ganglion
B. nasociliary nerve
C. short ciliary nerve
D. long ciliary nerve

44. Nearpoint-stress myopia is caused by a spasm of the 44.____

A. iris
B. zonula fibers
C. rectus tendon
D. ciliary muscle

45. Receptors located on the temporal side of the left retina are activated by light stimuli in the ______ half of the visual field and project into the ______ side of the brain. 45.____

A. right; left
B. left; right
C. right; right
D. left; left

46. Which of the following is LEAST likely to cause corneal opacities? 46.____

A. Phenytoin (Dilantin)
B. Amiodarone
C. Chloroquine
D. Tamoxifen

47. In the lacrimal gland, 47.____

A. ductules open into the conjunctiva at the upper margin of the upper tarsus
B. there is no true capsule
C. the palpebral section is larger than the orbital section
D. both the palpebral and orbital sections have ductules that open separately into the conjunctiva

48. Some rhodopsin is regenerated by the reaction of vitamin A with 48.____

A. opsin
B. transducin
C. scotopsin
D. phosphodiesterase

49. Which of the following does NOT induce cycloplegia? 49._____

A. Tropicamide
B. Cyclopentolate
C. Phenylephrine
D. Atropine

50. Which of the following is a major inhibitory neurotransmitter in the retina? 50._____

A. glutamate
B. glycine
C. acetylcholine
D. dopamine

KEY (CORRECT ANSWERS)

1. A	11. C	21. D	31. D	41. C
2. D	12. C	22. A	32. B	42. D
3. D	13. A	23. A	33. D	43. C
4. A	14. D	24. C	34. C	44. D
5. B	15. A	25. B	35. B	45. A
6. A	16. D	26. B	36. C	46. A
7. B	17. A	27. C	37. A	47. B
8. A	18. D	28. A	38. C	48. C
9. C	19. C	29. D	39. D	49. C
10. B	20. B	30. A	40. B	50. B

TEST 2

DIRECTIONS: Each question or incomplete statement is followed by several suggested answers or completions. Select the one that BEST answers the question or completes the statement. *PRINT THE LETTER OF THE CORRECT ANSWER IN THE SPACE AT THE RIGHT.*

1. The recession of the visual near point throughout life is due principally to 1.____

   A. atrophy of the ciliary body
   B. flattening of the cornea
   C. hardening of the lens
   D. open-angle glaucoma

2. Which of the following would MOST likely be a cause of severe afferent pupillary defect (Marcus Gunn pupil?) 2.____

   A. Retinal scarring
   B. Vitreous hemorrhage
   C. Optic neuritis
   D. Amblyopia

3. The majority of the ocular blood flow passes through the 3.____

   A. retina
   B. cornea
   C. choroid
   D. sclera

4. Which of the following is NOT a symptom of iritis? 4.____

   A. blurred vision
   B. photosensitivity
   C. papilledema
   D. inflamed blood vessels around the limbus

5. Horner's syndrome is a combination of each of the following, EXCEPT 5.____

   A. ptosis
   B. anhydrosis
   C. miosis
   D. strabismus

6. The lens develops embryologically from the 6.____

   A. optical vesicle
   B. neural crest cells
   C. mesencephalon
   D. surface ectoderm

7. Which of the following occurs LAST in the photoreceptor response to light? 7._____

   A. Reduction of cGMP molecules in the cell
   B. Bonding of metarhodopsin and transducin
   C. Bonding of transducin and GTP
   D. Separation of retinene and opsin

8. The sympathetic nerve supply to the lacrimal gland does NOT travel through the 8._____

   A. pterygopalatine ganglion
   B. maxillary nerve
   C. greater petrosal nerve
   D. zygomatic nerve

9. The chromophore involved in color vision is 9._____

   A. 11-*cis*-retinal
   B. GTP
   C. transducin
   D. metarhodopsin

10. Which of the following statements about benzalkonium chloride is FALSE? 10._____

   A. It is inactivated by calcium
   B. It is most effective in a slightly alkaline solution
   C. It decreases the permeability of bacterial cell walls
   D. It is often used as a preservative

11. Which of the following does NOT result from the remnants of the hyaloid vasculature? 11._____

   A. Bergmeister's papilla
   B. Persistent pupillary membrane
   C. Posterior lenticonus
   D. Mittendorf's dot

12. Angioid streaks involve breaks in the 12._____

   A. Choroid
   B. Bruch's membrane
   C. Macula
   D. Retinal pigment epithelium

13. The eye's "blind spot" corresponds to the 13._____

   A. macula lutea
   B. fovea centralis
   C. optic disk
   D. ora serrata

14. Which of the following occurs FIRST within the rods when they are stimulated by light? 14._____

   A. The membrane becomes hyperpolarized
   B. The rate of transmitter release declines
   C. The rhodopsin molecule absorbs light
   D. The inflow of sodium ions decreases

15. The Young-Helmholtz theory of color vision postulates 15.____

A. 3 different kinds of cones
B. 3 different kinds of rods
C. 2 means of sensory input from the retina
D. 3 different aspects combined in the perception of depth

16. Which of the following enters the orbit through the annulus of Zinn? 16.____

A. Inferior ophthalmic vein
B. Superior ophthalmic vein
C. Lacrimal nerve
D. Nasociliary nerve

17. Which of the following topical medications does NOT induce a myopic shift? 17.____

A. physostigmine
B. Echothiophate
C. pilocarpine
D. Atropine

18. In the oculomotor nuclear complex, the nucleus for each ______ supplies the ipsilateral muscle. 18.____

A. central caudal area
B. superior rectus
C. inferior oblique
D. medial rectus

19. Which of the following is found in higher concentrations in the aqueous humor than in plasma? 19.____

A. Ascorbic aid
B. Glucose
C. Lactic acid
D. Protein

20. The term "visual threshold" refers to the 20.____

A. degree to which the details and contours of objects can be perceived
B. rate at which visual stimuli can be presented and still be perceived as distinct
C. the shortest distance by which two lines can be separated and still be perceived as two lines
D. minimal amount of light that elicits a sensation of light

21. Which of the following statements about the inferior oblique is TRUE? 21.____

A. It is innervated by the superior division of the oculomotor nerve
B. It passes anteroposteriorly below the inferior rectus.
C. It arises from the lacrimal bone.
D. It elevates the eyeball

22. The neural connections that mediate visual reflexes are formed in the 22.____

A. hypothalamus
B. inferior colliculus
C. geniculate body
D. superior colliculus

23. The annulus of Zinn 23.____

A. is formed by a network of the long posterior ciliary arteries
B. supplies the macula
C. is formed at the sclera
D. supplies the intraorbital part of the optic nerve

24. Which of the following layers of the geniculate body receive input from the contralateral eye? 24.____

A. 1, 2, and 3
B. 1, 4, and 6
C. 2, 3, and 4
D. 4, 5, and 6

25. The optic nerve fibers from the upper retinal quadrants subserving vision in the lower half of the visual field terminate in the 25.____

A. lateral half of the lateral geniculate body
B. medial half of the lateral geniculate body
C. superior lip of the calcarine fissure
D. inferior lip of the calcarine fissure

26. The cells in the macular pigment epithelium, compared to those in the retinal pigment epithelium, 26.____

A. are shorter
B. are thinner
C. contain fewer villi
D. contain more melanosomes

27. Which of the following would NOT cause swelling in the optic disk? 27.____

A. Hypotony
B. Retrobulbar neuritis
C. Posterior uveitis
D. Occlusion of the central retinal vein

28. Which of the following is NOT known to cause or contribute to cataract? 28.____

A. Chlorpromazine (Thorazine)
B. Simvastatin
C. Ultraviolet light
D. Fluoxetine (Prozac)

29. ______ accounts for 90% of the total protein in the rods. 29.____

A. Rhodopsin
B. Phosphodiesterase
C. Transducin
D. Scotopsin

30. Axons of ganglion cells on the nasal portion of the brain cross over at the ______ to project to opposite side of the brain. 30.____

A. lacrimal gland
B. optic chiasm
C. suprachiasmatic nucleus
D. lateral portion of the retina

31. ______ eye movements function to seek out visual targets. 31.____

A. Pursuit
B. Saccadic
C. Convergence
D. Vestibular

32. Which of the following occurs during accommodation? 32.____

A. Sympathetic outflow to the ciliary body increases
B. Tension in the suspensatory ligament in increased
C. Tension in the lens capsule increases
D. The refractive power of the lens increases

33. Which of the following would be LEAST effective on Cytomegalovi-rus (CMV) retinitis? 33.____

A. Ganciclovir
B. Acyclovir
C. Cidofovir
D. Rifabutin

34. The ______ is the point within the eye through which the light rays from an object pass without refraction ^ 34.____

A. blind spot
B. nodal point
C. fovea
D. vitreous humor

35. The superior oblique muscle is supplied by the ______ cranial nerve on its upper surface. 35.____

A. third
B. fourth
C. fifth
D. sixth

36. Visual information processing in the retina involve the formation of three images. The second image is formed in the ______ cells. 36.____

A. horizontal
B. bipolar
C. amacrine
D. ganglion

37. The principal neurons of the dorsal lateral geniculate body send their axons to a region of the occipital cortex known variously by each of the following names, EXCEPT 37.____

A. Bordmann's area
B. the calcarine cortex
C. V4
D. the striate cortex

38. The largest branch of the ophthalmic nerve is the ______ nerve. 38.____

A. frontal
B. lacrimal
C. zygomatic
D. nasociliary

39. Which of the following statements about the fovea is FALSE? 39.____

A. It has no retinal vessels
B. It has no short-wavelength cones
C. It is covered in part by the macula lutea
D. It is a very thick retinal layer

40. Which of the following denotes a parasympathetic ganglion? 40.____

A. Otic
B. Stellate
C. Gasserian
D. Ciliary

41. Since rods outnumber cones in the human eye, the overall ratio of convergence of the photoreceptors through bipolar cells onto ganglion cells is, rod to cone, about ______: 1 41.____

A. 5
B. 18
C. 50
D. 105

42. Symptoms of vitamin A deficiency include each of the following, EXCEPT 42.____

A. sterile corneal ulceration
B. night blindness
C. palsy of extraocular muscles
D. Bitot's spots

43. During retinal metabolism, 43.____

A. oxygen demand is met by the central retinal artery
B. aerobic metabolism is predominant
C. lactate is accumulated
D. insulin is required for the uptake of glucose

44. Which of the following structures is/are posterior to the Meibomian glands? 44.____

A. Glands of Krause
B. Glands of Zeis
C. Glands of Moll
D. Muscle of Riolan

45. Axonal processes of the photoreceptors extend toward the ______ layer , where they establish contacts with bipolar cells and horizontal cells. 45.____

A. outer plexiform
B. inner plexiform
C. outer nuclear
D. pigment epithelium

46. Which of the following types of nerve fibers synapse in the ciliary ganglion? 46.____

A. parasympathetic oculomotor nerve
B. sympathetic carotid plexus
C. abducent nerve
D. nasociliary nerve

47. Which of the following would be associated with a lesion in the right medial longitudinal fasciculus (MLF)? 47.____

A. Problems with supraversion
B. Impaired right adduction
C. Problems with convergence
D. Impaired left adduction

48. Pilocarpine is contraindicated in cases of ______ glaucoma. 48.____

A. subacute angle closure
B. aphakic
C. malignant
D. pseudoexfoliation

49. Embryologically, the ciliary epithelium is derived from the 49.____

A. surface ectoderm
B. optic cup
C. neural crest cells
D. blastoderm

50. Floaters-also known as "muscae volitantes"- which sometimes interfere with vision, can be caused by 50.____

A. glaucoma
B. color deficiency
C. cataract
D. vitreous detachment

KEY (CORRECT ANSWERS)

1. C	11. C	21. D	31. B	41. D
2. C	12. B	22. D	32. D	42. C
3. C	13. C	23. C	33. B	43. C
4. C	14. C	24. B	34. B	44. A
5. D	15. A	25. B	35. B	45. A
6. D	16. D	26. A	36. B	46. A
7. D	17. D	27. B	37. C	47. B
8. C	18. D	28. D	38. A	48. C
9. A	19. A	29. A	39. D	49. B
10. C	20. D	30. B	40. A	50. D

TEST 3

DIRECTIONS: Each question or incomplete statement is followed by several suggested answers or completions. Select the one that BEST answers the question or completes the statement. *PRINT THE LETTER OF THE CORRECT ANSWER IN THE SPACE AT THE RIGHT.*

1. ______ eye movements are adjustments that occur in response to stimuli initiated in the semicircular canals. 1.____

   A. Convergence
   B. Vestibular
   C. Saccadic
   D. Pursuit

2. Which of the following occurs FIRST in the photoreceptor response to light? 2.____

   A. Metarhodopsin II cleaves to transducin
   B. Phosphodiesterase cleaves to cGMP molecules
   C. 11-*cis*-retinal changes shape and converts to trans-retinal
   D. The sodium ion channel is shut down

3. Which of the following is NOT innervated by the oculomotor nerve? 3.____

   A. superior rectus
   B. inferior oblique
   C. medial rectus
   D. lateral rectus

4. Each of the following arises embryologically from the surface ectoderm, EXCEPT the 4.____

   A. sclera
   B. lens
   C. conjunctival epithelium
   D. lacrimal gland

5. At the extreme periphery of the visual field, there is a zone seen only by the eye on that side. This area is sometimes called the 5.____

   A. centralateral blind spot
   B. monocular crescent
   C. temporal scotoma
   D. hemifield

6. In the visual pathway, ganglion cells axons project a spatial representation of each retina onto the 6.____

   A. geniculate body
   B. trochlear nucleus
   C. Edinger-Westphal nucleus
   D. complex cells of the visual cortex

7. The density of nerve endings on the cornea is about ______ that of the epidermis. 7.____

A. half
B. twice
C. 10 times
D. 300 times

8. For practical purposes, light rays from an object that strike a lens more than ______ feet away are considered to be parallel 8.____

A. 6
B. 12
C. 20
D. 100

9. The superior branch of the oculomotor nerve supplies the 9.____

A. superior rectus
B. medial rectus
C. levator inferioris
D. inferior oblique

10. The direct light reflex of the pupil can occur in association with 10.____

A. a complete ipsilateral third nerve palsy
B. a lesion of the ipsilateral ciliary ganglion
C. the topical application of phenyephrine
D. the transaction of the ipsilateral optic nerve

11. The outer segment of a human photoreceptor is completely shed and regenerated in a cycle of 11.____

A. 24-48 hours
B. 3 to 8 days
C. 9-13 days
D. 25-37 days

12. The ciliary body contains about ______ ciliary processes. 12.____

A. 12
B. 70
C. 150
D. 320

13. Which of the following has a mydriatic effect? 13.____

A. Neostigmine
B. Carbachol
C. Echothiophate
D. Phenylephrine

14. Which of the following would NOT cause an increase in intraocular pressure? 14.____

A. Coughing
B. Pupil dilation
C. Drinking alcohol
D. Normal blinking

15. The pathway for the light reflex passes from the pre-tectal region to the 15.____

A. Edinger-Westphal nuclei
B. zonule
C. ciliary ganglion
D. nodal point

16. Which of the following statements about the sodium ion channels in the outer segments of the rods is FALSE? 16.____

A. The receptor potential is hyperpolarized
B. They are open in the dark.
C. Current flows from the inner to the outer segment.
D. Current flows to the synaptic ending of the photoreceptor

17. A palsy of the left fourth nerve can cause 17.____

A. diplopia with head tilt to he right
B. left ocular hyperdeviation on looking right
C. torsional diplopia
D. head tilt to the left

18. A minimum angle of resolution (MAR) is LEAST likely to be affected by the 18.____

A. brightness of the stimuli
B. state of retinal adaptation
C. regularity of the borders on stimuli
D. position of the stimuli on the retina

19. Each of the following would be a possible suspected cause of an iritis or uveitis, EXCEPT 19.____

A. tuberculosis
B. arthritis
C. psoriasis
D. ankylosing spondylitis

20. The first branch of the internal carotid artery after it enters the sub-arachnoid space is the _______ artery. 20.____

A. posterior communicating
B. middle cerebral
C. ophthalmic
D. anterior choroidal

21. A retinal ganglion cell with an on-center receptive field will fire a high frequency burst of action potentials when: 21.____

A. the center of its receptive field is fully illuminated by a concentrated spot of light
B. the center of its receptive field is in darkness and its surround is fully illuminated
C. both the center of its receptive field and surround are fully illuminated
D. glutamate released from the cone excites the bipolar cells

22. The perception that nearby objects move more quickly than distant objects is the result of a phenomenon known as 22.____

A. stereopsis
B. motion parallax
C. occlusion
D. retinal disparity

23. Looking left involves an increased contraction of the 23.____

A. right superior rectus
B. right inferior oblique
C. left medial rectus
D. left lateral rectus

24. Which of the following ophthalmic drugs is LEAST likely to cause ptosis? 24.____

A. Guanethidine
B. Thymoxamine
C. Pilocarpine
D. Carbachol

25. Which of the following is LEAST likely to cause an opacity of the lens? 25.____

A. Tamoxifen
B. Aspirin
C. Chlorpromazine
D. Amiodarone

26. Each of the following proteins found in the tear of the normal eye have antibacterial properties, EXCEPT 26.____

A. lymphokines
B. lactoferrin
C. betalysin
D. lysozyme

27. Each of the following is an effect of histamines on the eye, EXCEPT 27.____

A. smooth muscle spasm
B. increased mucus production
C. dilation of conjunctival capillaries
D. lowered prostaglandin production

28. In the lacrimal gland tissue, the 28.____

    A. histology is similar to the salivary glands
    B. oculomotor nerve supplies the parasympathetic innervation
    C. blood supply comes from a branch of the facial artery
    D. gland of Wolfring is located between the conjunctiva and sclera

29. Rhodopsin 29.____

    A. is variably sensitive to purple light
    B. is produced on the outer segments of rods
    C. is most sensitive to blue-green light
    D. does not regenerate when the eyes are closed

30. Which of the following will affect the pupil size, while having no effect on lens accommodation? 30.____

    A. Echothiophate
    B. Tropicamide
    C. Phenylephrine
    D. Latanoprost

31. Which of the following statements about the lacrimal gland is FALSE? 31.____

    A. Its parasympathetic nerve supply comes from the deep petrosal nerve
    B. It is visible when the upper lid is turned inside out
    C. Its palpebral part is smaller than its orbital part
    D. It is a C-shaped structure

32. The only cells that secrete acetylcholine in the retina are ______ cells. 32.____

    A. amacrine
    B. bipolar
    C. ganglion
    D. horizontal

33. Of the following, the "extraspectral" color is 33.____

    A. red
    B. purple
    C. green
    D. blue

34. About 7% of the total ocular blood flow is received by the 34.____

    A. ciliary body
    B. retina
    C. choroid
    D. sclera

35. Light-near dissociation can be caused by lesions in each of the following regions, EXCEPT the 35.____

A. occipital cortex
B. ciliary ganglion
C. pre-tectal nucleus
D. optic nerve

36. Which of the following structures do(es) NOT originate embryologi-cally from neural crest cells? 36.____

A. Corneal endothelium
B. Corneal stroma
C. Zonules
D. Choroidal melanocytes

37. Which of the following is NOT involved in color vision? 37.____

A. Visual cortex area V8
B. Geniculate layer
C. M pathway
D. P pathway

38. The neural elements of the retina are bound together by glial cells known as ______ cells. 38.____

A. midget bipolar
B. Muller
C. horizontal
D. amacrine

39. The vortex veins 39.____

A. are more easily observable in dark-complected, dark-eyed subjects
B. number about 6 in each eye
C. drain the choroid
D. drain the retina

40. Each cone in the fovea has a ______ cell connecting it to a single ganglion cell. 40.____

A. flat bipolar
B. rid bipolar
C. horizontal
D. midget bipolar

41. ______ phenomenon is associated with optic neuritis. 41.____

A. Pulfrich's
B. Aubert's
C. Raynaud's
D. Troller's

42. The biochemical antioxidant zeaxanthin is 42.____

A. heavier than lutein
B. found within the retinal pigment epithelium
C. more concentrated in cones than rods
D. often used as a preservative in topical ophthalmic drugs

43. Bruch's membrane is 43.____

A. absent at the fovea
B. about 5 mm thick
C. secreted by the retinal pigment epithelium
D. penetrated by the choriocapillaries

44. In the tear film, 44.____

A. the inner mucous layer is formed by the conjunctiva
B. the main immunoglobulin is Ig G
C. mucous layer deficiencies are detected with Schirmer tear test
D. the aqueous layer is produced mainly by the lacrimal gland

45. Light adaptation is nearly maximal at about ______ minutes. 45.____

A. 5
B. 10
C. 20
D. 40

46. Each of the following bones covers the nasolacrimal duct, EXCEPT the 46.____

A. medial turbinate
B. inferior turbinate
C. ethmoid
D. maxillary

47. In the _______, neural fibers from the nasal half of one retina and temporal half of another synapse on the cells whose axons form the geniculocalcarine tract. 47.____

A. optic chiasm
B. optic tract
C. visual cortex
D. geniculate body

48. A lesion that interrupts the optic chiasm will cause blindness in 48.____

A. opposite sides of the visual fields
B. half of one visual field
C. one eye
D. both eyes

49. A patient had a Marcus Gunn pupil, but now has normal pupillary reaction to light. Which of the following may explain this? 49.____

A. There is ischemic optic neuropathy in both eyes.
B. A bilateral papilledema has developed.
C. The affected eye was treated with cyclopentolate
D. The patient had a cataract removed.

50. Accommodation is NOT 50.____

A. regulated with the help of chromatic aberrations
B. associated with an increased curvature on the anterior surface of the lens
C. mandatory for the perception of stereopsis
D. dependent on the elasticity of the capsule

KEY (CORRECT ANSWERS)

1. B	11. C	21. A	31. B	41. A
2. C	12. B	22. B	32. A	42. C
3. D	13. D	23. D	33. B	43. C
4. A	14. C	24. C	34. A	44. A
5. B	15. A	25. B	35. A	45. A
6. A	16. A	26. A	36. C	46. A
7. D	17. C	27. D	37. C	47. D
8. C	18. C	28. A	38. B	48. A
9. A	19. C	29. C	39. C	49. A
10. C	20. C	30. C	40. D	50. C

TEST 4

DIRECTIONS: Each question or incomplete statement is followed by several suggested answers or completions. Select the one that BEST answers the question or completes the statement. *PRINT THE LETTER OF THE CORRECT ANSWER IN THE SPACE AT THE RIGHT.*

1. "Yoke muscle" pairs in the eye include each of the following, EXCEPT the 1.____

   A. left inferior oblique and right superior rectus
   B. left superior rectus and right inferior rectus
   C. left lateral rectus and right medial rectus
   D. left inferior rectus and right superior oblique

2. Approximately ______% of the cones in the retina lie outside the central 5 degrees of the macula. 2.____

   A. 10
   B. 30
   C. 60
   D. 90

3. The capillary plexus in the choroid, and not the retinal vessels, generally supplies the 3.____

   A. bipolar cells
   B. ganglion cells
   C. photoreceptors
   D. amacrine cells

4. Which of the following is a copper deposit that may be found in Descemet's membrane? 4.____

   A. Ferry's line
   B. Arcus senilis
   C. Kayser-Fleischer ring
   D. Hudson-Stahl's line

5. The cell membranes of cones contain 5.____

   A. disks, but no saccules
   B. saccules, but no disks
   C. both saccules and disks
   D. neither saccules nor disks

6. Non-steroidal anti-inflammatory drugs (NSAIDs) such as diclofenac 6.____

   A. are used to treat corneal surface pain
   B. are contraindicated with asthma patients
   C. decrease intraocular pressure
   D. often require the use of fluoroquinolone as a prophylactic

7. In the outer plexiform, ______ cells connect receptor cells to one another. 7.____

   A. horizontal
   B. rod bipolar
   C. amacrine
   D. flat bipolar

8. Which of the following nerves does NOT carry parasympathetic impulses to the lacrimal gland? 8.____

   A. greater petrosal
   B. superior branch of the oculomotor
   C. deep petrosal
   D. zygomaticotemporal

9. Current that leaves the photoreceptor's inner segment is carried largely by ______ ions. 9.____

   A. magnesium
   B. sodium
   C. calcium
   D. potassium

10. The *c*-wave of an electroretinogram is generated in the 10.____

    A. rods
    B. inner plexiform
    C. pigment epithelium
    D. cones

11. The lens 11.____

    A. has a uniform refractive index
    B. is innervated by the short ciliary nerve
    C. does not grow after birth
    D. has a larger radius of curvature in front (anteriorly) than in the back (posteriorly)

12. The axons from the lateral geniculate neurons terminate at pyramidal cells in layer ______ of the visual cortex. 12.____

    A. 2
    B. 3
    C. 4
    D. 5

13. The short ciliar,y nerves trave ______ between the sclera and the choroid. 13.____

    A. anteriorly
    B. posteriorly
    C. medially
    D. laterally

14. Which of the following is NOT an effect of direct-acting cholinergic agonists? 14.____

    A. Traction on peripheral retina
    B. Mydriasis

C. Decrease in zonular tension
D. Increased depth focus

15. Which of the following topical medications is contraindicated in iritis? 15.____

A. Betaxolol
B. Atropine
C. Pilocarpine
D. Acetazolamide

16. The retinal ganglion cells known as Y cells 16.____

A. have small axons
B. are sensitive to slow motion
C. conduct impulses slowly
D. have a large receptive field

17. The long ciliary nerve 17.____

A. enters the eyeball at the equator
B. contains parasympathetic nerve fibers
C. contains sensory fibers from the cornea
D. branches from the supraorbital nerve

18. Dark adaptation is nearly maximal at about ______ minutes. 18.____

A. 5
B. 10
C. 20
D. 40

19. Within the iris, 19.____

A. eye color is determined by parasympathetic innervations
B. the constrictor muscle receives sympathetic innervation
C. eye color is determined by melanocytes in the stroma
D. there is pigmented epithelium on the anterior surface

20. The outer segments of rods and cones consist of 20.____

A. cell nuclei
B. mitochondria
C. horizontal cells
D. modified cilia

21. Which of the following will decrease tear osmolality? 21.____

A. Widening palpebral fissures
B. Punctal stenosis
C. Meibomitis
D. Decreased corneal sensation

22. In papilledema, 22.____

A. eye movements are painful
B. the condition is usually unilateral
C. an initial effect is an enlarged blind spot
D. there is usually an altered pupillary response

23. The ______ passes through the ring-like tendon known as the trochlea, in the nasal orbit. 23.____

A. A medial rectus
B. superior rectus
C. superior oblique
D. inferior oblique

24. Which of the following statements about ocular circulation is FALSE? 24.____

A. The retinal blood vessels dilate during hypoxia
B. Normally, the choroidal flood flow is about ten times that of the flow to a comparable volume of the brain's gray matter.
C. About 25% of the eye's total blood supply goes to the retina
D. A rise in arterial CO_2 pressure produces a rise in retinal blood flow

25. Which of the following statements about lutein is TRUE? 25.____

A. It is found in the retinal pigment epithelium
B. It is water-soluble
C. It shields the eye from yellow light
D. It is dispersed throughout the retina

26. Corneal sensation is 26.____

A. uniform throughout
B. greatest at the apex and diminishes toward the limbus
C. greatest at the limbus and diminishes toward the apex
D. greater in the nasal than the temporal half

27. The levator superioris palpebris opposes the action of the 27.____

A. frontalis
B. orbicularis oculi
C. inferior oblique
D. superior rectus

28. The ocular muscles are innervated by each of the following nerves, EXCEPT the 28.____

A. oculomotor
B. trochlear
C. lacrimal
D. abducens

29. The contraction of the superior rectus and inferior oblique muscles, accompanied by an equal relaxation of the of the inferior rectus and superior oblique muscles, results in 29.____

A. abduction
B. supraduction
C. extorsion
D. infraduction

30. A lesion that interrupts one optic tract will cause blindness in 30.____

A. one eye
B. both eyes
C. half of one visual field
D. half of both visual fields

31. Which of the following passes through the inferior orbital fissure? 31.____

A. Orbital branch of middle meningeal artery
B. Frontal nerve
C. Infraorbital vein
D. Recurrent branch of lacrimal artery

32. Important monocular clues to distance include each of the following, EXCEPT 32.____

A. retinal disparity
B. size
C. perspective
D. occlusion

33. Which of the following is an accessory nucleus of the third oculomotor nerve that relays pre-ganglionic parasympathetics to the eye, which constrict the pupil and accommodate the lens. 33.____

A. trochlear nucleus
B. epiganglion
C. pretectum
D. Edinger-Westphal nucleus

34. Which of the following is NOT embrologically derived from the neural crest cells? 34.____

A. Ciliary muscles
B. Lens
C. Corneal endothelium
D. Sclera

35. Which of the following drugs will increase aqueous secretion? 35.____

A. Pilocarpine
B. Albuterol
C. Methazolamide (Neptazane)
D. Digoxin

36. Which of the following statements about the ciliary body is FALSE? 36.____

A. It extends 8mm beyond the corneoscleral junction
B. It receives blood from the short posterior ciliary arteries.

C. It consists of the pars plicata and the pars plana.
D. It produces aqueous humor.

37. Vitamin ______ deficiency is a cause of optic neuropathy. 37.____

A. B_1
B. B_3
C. B_6
D. B_{12}

38. A patient is blind, but the pupillary light reflex is intact. It would be safe to say that the cause is a lesion somewhere behind the 38.____

A. geniculocalcarine tract
B. optic chiasm
C. optic nerve
D. optic tract

39. Of the following, esotropia is most likely to be caused by a palsy of the 39.____

A. medial rectus
B. lateral rectus
C. inferior oblique
D. superior oblique

40. The pupil may respond to light stimulus if the 40.____

A. sympathetic system is not functioning
B. optic nerve is severed
C. cholinergic system is blocked
D. pretectal nucleus is damaged

41. Each of the following statements about corneal penetration of a topical drug is true, EXCEPT that the penetration is 41.____

A. decreased if the drug is made more hydrophilic
B. decreased if the subject blinks more frequently
C. increased if the epithelium is removed
D. increased if the intraocular pressure is reduced

42. The normal rate of blinking is considered to be about ______ per minute. 42.____

A. 2
B. 5
C. 12
D. 20

43. Within the retina, the responses of each of the following is hyperpolar-izing, EXCEPT the 43.____

A. rods
B. cones
C. amacrine cells
D. horizontal cells

44. Which of the following would be caused by a lesion of the trigeminal nerve? 44.____

A. Ectropion of the lower eyelid
B. Ptosis of the upper eyelid
C. Mydriasis
D. Decreased corneal sensation

45. Descemet's membrane 45.____

A. regenerates when damaged
B. pumps fluid from the cornea
C. is composed of collagen fibrils
D. lies just under the endothelium

46. Mydriatic drugs act by imitating the action of 46.____

A. norepinephrine
B. beta carotenes
C. acetylcholine
D. opsin

47. Which of the following is NOT supplied by the short ciliary nerves? 47.____

A. Ciliary muscle
B. Sphincter pupillae
C. Lens
D. Dilator pupillae

48. The anti-glaucoma agent physostigmine may involve each of the following, EXCEPT 48.____

A. twitching of the eyelids
B. conjunctival vasoconstriction
C. decreased intraocular pressure
D. accommodative spasm

49. Which of the following is more concentrated in the tear than in the serum? 49.____

A. immunoglobulin G
B. potassium
C. glucose
D. sodium

50. Acute, or closed-angle, glaucoma 50.____

A. involves corneal opacity that is caused by inflammatory cells in the anterior chamber
B. can be treated with acetazolamide
C. is usually bilateral
D. affects a high number of younger patients

KEY (CORRECT ANSWERS)

1.	B	11.	D	21.	B	31.	C	41.	D
2.	D	12.	C	22.	C	32.	A	42.	C
3.	C	13.	A	23.	C	33.	D	43.	C
4.	C	14.	B	24.	C	34.	B	44.	D
5.	B	15.	C	25.	D	35.	B	45.	B
6.	A	16.	D	26.	B	36.	A	46.	A
7.	A	17.	D	27.	B	37.	A	47.	C
8.	B	18.	C	28.	C	38.	D	48.	B
9.	D	19.	C	29.	B	39.	B	49.	B
10.	C	20.	D	30.	D	40.	A	50.	B

TEST 5

DIRECTIONS: Each question or incomplete statement is followed by several suggested answers or completions. Select the one that BEST answers the question or completes the statement. *PRINT THE LETTER OF THE CORRECT ANSWER IN THE SPACE AT THE RIGHT.*

1. In the photoreceptors, 1._____

   A. nutrients are received from choroidal circulation
   B. the inner segment has a smaller diameter than the outer segment
   C. the outer segments are oriented with their short axes toward the pupil
   D. the synaptic terminals are located in the inner plexiform layer

2. Ophthalmoscopic examination is of great value in the diagnosis and evaluation of diabetes mellitus, hypertension, and other diseases because 2._____

   A. pathology of the eye is one of the first indicators of these diseases
   B. the retina is the only place in the body where arterioles are readily visible
   C. these diseases usually involve visual problems
   D. these diseases usually involve neovascularization

3. Which of the following does NOT affect pupil size? 3._____

   A. Physical activity
   B. Iris color
   C. Refractive error
   D. Fatigue

4. In the lateral geniculate, the parvocellular layers carry the signals for each of the following, EXCEPT 4._____

   A. fine depth
   B. shape
   C. color
   D. detection of movement

5. In the inner plexiform, ______ cells connect ganglion cells to one another. 5._____

   A. horizontal
   B. amacrine
   C. glial
   D. Müller

6. Which of the following subcortical structures is NOT known to be activated by visual stimuli? 6._____

   A. caudate nucleus
   B. amygdala
   C. inferior colliculus
   D. superior colliculus

7. Which of the following terms denotes a red color weakness in the visual system? 7.____

   A. Tritanopia
   B. Tritanomaly
   C. Protanopia
   D. Protanomaly

8. The parasympathetic innervation of the lacrimal gland branches from the supersalivary nucleus. Which of the following structures does it then pass through FIRST? 8.____

   A. Greater petrosal nerve
   B. Nervus intermedius
   C. Pterygopalatine fossa
   D. Zygomaticotemporal nerve

9. The zonules are embryologically derived from the 9.____

   A. ectoderm
   B. mesoderm
   C. tertiary vitreous
   D. hyaloid artery

10. Which of the following muscles does NOT lower the eyebrow? 10.____

   A. Orbicularis oculi
   B. Procerus
   C. Corrugator supercilii
   D. Frontalis

11. The scotopic visual apparatus is capable of determining the 11.____

   A. small details in objects
   B. colors of objects
   C. boundaries of objects
   D. presence of an object under reduced illumination

12. The layer of the cornea that serves primarily to protect it from injury is the 12.____

   A. Bowman's membrane
   B. Descemet's membrane
   C. stroma
   D. epithelium

13. On viewing an object, the impulses set up in both retinas combine at the cortex to form a single image. This is known as 13.____

   A. stereopsis
   B. fixation
   C. focus
   D. fusion

14. The lens capsule is composed mostly of 14.____

A. type I collagen
B. type IV collagen
C. alpha-crystallin
D. gamma-crystallin

15. Macular sparing, or loss of peripheral vision with intact macular vision, is commonly seen with lesions of the 15.____

A. optic chiasm
B. optic nerve
C. optic tract
D. visual cortex

16. A patient's pupillary response to light is absent, but response to accommodation is normal. This phenomenon is known as 16.____

A. Horner's syndrome
B. Lowe's phenomenon
C. Argyll Robertson pupil
D. Bell's phenomenon

17. Which of the following passes through the superior orbital fissure? 17.____

A. Nasociliary nerve
B. Zygomatic nerve
C. Infraorbital nerve
D. Parasympathetics to lacrimal gland

18. Retinal vascularization typically begins at the ______ month of gestation. 18.____

A. 2nd
B. 4th
C. 6th
D. 8th

19. Within the retina, ______ cells produce depolarizing potentials and spikes that may act as generator potential for the propagated spikes produced in other cells. 19.____

A. Müller
B. amacrine
C. midget bipolar
D. saccule

20. Which of the following is involved in vergence eye movements? 20.____

A. Burst neurons
B. Accommodation
C. Conjugate movement
D. Sympathetic pathway

21. A topical eyedrop will have a decreased penetration rate if it 21.____

A. contains liposomes
B. has a pH of exactly 7.4
C. produces a tearing reflex
D. contains preservative

22. The most common cause of vertical ocular misalignment is paralysis of the ______ nerve. 22.____

A. oculomotor
B. optic
C. trigeminal
D. trochlear

23. The "ocular blood barrier," analogous to the blood-brain barrier, is contained within the capillary walls of the 23.____

A. iris
B. choroid
C. ciliary body
D. retina

24. Which of the following is NOT a possible effect of pilocarpine? 24.____

A. Increased lens thickness
B. Increased zonular tension
C. Ciliary body contraction
D. Greater permeability of iris vessels

25. Timolol solution 25.____

A. should not be used in conjunction with latanoprost
B. may cause mydriasis
C. is a selective beta-blocker
D. acts upon the eye for about 6 to 8 hours

26. During the pupillary light reflex, the Edinger-Westphal nuclei are activated by the 26.____

A. trochlear nuclei
B. ciliary ganglion
C. pretectal nuclei
D. suprachiasmatic nucleus

27. Which of the following types of cells is NOT contained in the inner plexiform? 27.____

A. Ganglion cells
B. Photoreceptors
C. Bipolar cells
D. Müller cells

28. Which of the following statements about intraocular pressure is FALSE? 28.____

A. It is underestimated in highly myopic patients if measured with the indentation method
B. It shows a higher daily variability in glaucoma patients
C. It is often overestimated in patients with a thick cornea
D. It is higher in the evening than in the morning

29. The fovea is located ______ to the optic disk 29.____

A. medially and slightly inferiorly
B. temporally and slightly inferiorly
C. slightly to either side, superiorly
D. medially and slightly superiorly

30. Which of the following bones forms the optic canal? 30.____

A. Frontal
B. Lacrimal
C. Temporal
D. Lesser wing of the sphenoid

31. Which of the following medications may create a pigmentation in the conjunctiva? 31.____

A. Acetazolamide
B. Dipivefrin
C. Betaxolol
D. Pilocarpine

32. The inferior oblique muscle 32.____

A. passes between the superior rectus and the eyeball on the way to insertion
B. has the longest tendon of all the extraocular muscles
C. arises from the anterolateral orbital floor
D. is innervated by the inferior division of the oculomotor nerve

33. Each of the following immunoglobulins is found in the tear, EXCEPT 33.____

A. A
B. D
C. E
D. M

34. Each of the following reactions involved in the photoreceptor mechanism can occur independent of light, EXCEPT the 34.____

A. conversion of 11-cis-retinal into trans-retinal
B. formation of metarhodopsin II
C. regeneration of rhodopsin
D. binding of transducin to GTP

35. A contraction of the medial rectus, accompanied by an equal relaxation of the lateral re tus, results in 35.____

A. infraduction
B. intorsion
C. supraduction
D. adduction

36. In anterior uveitis, each of the following is true, EXEPT that 36.____

A. the irregularity of the pupil is due to adhesions between the lens and the cornea
B. the condition worsens when reading
C. it is associated with ankylosing spondylitis
D. glaucoma may be a complication

37. Which of the following statements about scotopic vision is FALSE? 37.____

A. It has poor acuity.
B. It is more sensitive to shorter light wavelengths.
C. It involves high foveal sensitivity.
D. There is no color vision involved.

38. The FIRST symptom of presbyopia is typically 38.____

A. blurred vision after looking away from a near distance
B. eyestrain while reading
C. diplopia
D. blurred print while reading

39. The inhibition of the retina's response to central illumination by an increase in the surround is known as ______ inhibition. 39.____

A. medial
B. afferent
C. divergent
D. efferent

40. The glands of ______ are responsible for secreting the mucous component of the tear film. 40.____

A. Krause
B. Wolfring
C. Moll
D. Zeis

41. The ciliary ganglion is found 41.____

A. 1 mm in front of the annulus of Zinn
B. near the floor of the orbit
C. between the lateral orbital wall and the lateral rectus muscle
D. above the ophthalmic artery

42. About ______ % of the ciliary body's innervation is parasympathetic. 42.____

A. 5
B. 40
C. 66
D. 97

43. Along the optic nerve, the 43.____

A. intracranial segment is the longest
B. intraorbital segment has the most variable length
C. intracanalicular segment is the longest
D. intraocular segment is the shortest

44. ______ nystagmus is a consequence of the relative motion of the visual field. 44.____

A. Jerk
B. Optokinetic
C. Pendular
D. Vestibular

45. Which of the following statements about the inferior oblique is FALSE? 45.____

A. It runs above the inferior rectus
B. It inserts to the sclera near the macula
C. It arises from the lateral orbital floor
D. It has the shortest tendon of all extraocular muscles

46. Which of the following is a selective betal-blocker? 46.____

A. Levobunolol
B. Betaxolol
C. Timolol
D. Carteolol

47. Which of the following may cause increased intraocular pressure in a normal eye? 47.____

A. Respiratory obstruction
B. Retrobulbar block
C. Hypoxia
D. Atropine

48. The sympathetic nerve supply to the iris travels through the 48.____

A. annulus of Zinn
B. cavernous sinus
C. orbicularis oculis
D. ora serrata

49. The lesser wing of the sphenoid bone provides an attachment for each of the following muscles, EXCEPT the 49.____

A. inferior oblique
B. superior rectus
C. superior oblique
D. levator palpebrae superioris

50. If the visual axis of one eye is directed at an object so that the image is positioned on the fovea, the eye is said to ______ the object. 50.____

A. fixate
B. formulate
C. focus
D. fuse

KEY (CORRECT ANSWERS)

1. A	11. D	21. C	31. B	41. A
2. B	12. A	22. D	32. D	42. D
3. C	13. D	23. D	33. B	43. D
4. D	14. B	24. B	34. A	44. B
5. B	15. D	25. B	35. D	45. A
6. C	16. C	26. C	36. A	46. B
7. D	17. A	27. B	37. C	47. C
8. B	18. B	28. D	38. A	48. B
9. C	19. B	29. B	39. B	49. A
10. D	20. B	30. D	40. B	50. A

EXAMINATION SECTION
TEST 1

DIRECTIONS: Each question or incomplete statement is followed by several suggested answers or completions. Select the one that BEST answers the question or completes the statement. *PRINT THE LETTER OF THE CORRECT ANSWER IN THE SPACE AT THE RIGHT.*

1. Which of the following compounds is the immediate source of the oxygen produced by photosynthesis? 1____

   A. Water
   B. Carbon dioxide
   C. Carbon monoxide
   D. Chlorophyll
   E. Magnesium oxide

2. Synthesis of glycogen from lactate in rat kidney cells requires the participation of enzymes localized in which of the following compartments? 2____

   I. Cytosol
   II. Mitochondria
   III. Peroxisomes

   The CORRECT answer is:

   A. I *only*
   B. II *only*
   C. III *only*
   D. I, II
   E. I, II, III

3. An *E. coli* mutant *(pol A)* with greatly reduced DNA polymerase I activity would be defective in DNA 3____

   A. endonucleolytic activity
   B. transcription
   C. excision repair
   D. unwinding
   E. recombination

4. Which of the following statements about operons is CORRECT? 4____

   A. Operons always contain at least three genes.
   B. Operons sometimes contain more than one promoter.
   C. Some eukaryotic genes are organized into operons.
   D. In an operon, both strands of the DNA are transcribed.
   E. In *E. coli,* operons frequently contain multiple copies of the same gene.

5. To study experimentally the movement of material across the intestinal epithelium, the lumen of the small intestine is filled with an electron-dense protein such as ferritin. When the tissue is subsequently fixed, sectioned, and examined using an electron microscope, the protein is found in small vesicles within the intestinal epithelial cells at the luminal surface. The protein is not found in the spaces between the cells. 5____
   The BEST explanation of this observation is that

   A. protein that penetrates between the cells is rapidly washed out by fluid flowing from the intestinal lumen toward blood vessels
   B. protein that penetrates between the cells is rapidly taken up by the cells into cytoplasmic vesicles
   C. protein does not penetrate between the cells because of tight junctions

D. the protein diffuses into the cells faster than it can penetrate through the functional complexes
E. only the protein that enters the cytoplasm of the cells is preserved during the preparation of the cells for microscopy

6. Polysaccharides of the plant cell are synthesized MAINLY in 6_____

A. the endoplasmic reticulum
B. the cytosol
C. the plasma membrane
D. dictyosomes
E. amyloplasts

7. *coli* moves in aqueous media by using which of the following? 7_____

A. Dynein B. Tubulin C. Actin
D. Flagellin E. Myosin

8. The binding of a ligand to a cell-surface hormone receptor is MOST analogous to the 8_____

A. formation of helical domains in a globular protein
B. hybridization of two single-stranded DNA molecules to form a helical duplex
C. assembly of phospholipids into a micelle
D. association of monomers into a multimeric complex
E. interaction of an enzyme with an allosteric effector

Questions 9-18.

DIRECTIONS: Each group of questions below consists of five lettered headings followed by a list of numbered phrases or sentences. For each numbered phrase or sentence, select the one heading that is MOST closely related to it. One heading may be used once, more than once, or not at all.

Questions 9-13 refer to the following enzymes.

A. Helicase
B. 3' → 5' exonuclease
C. Ligase
D. Topoisomerase II
E. Primase

9. Catalyzes double-strand cuts to facilitate unwinding of DNA. 9_____

10. Enhances separation of DNA strands during replication. 10_____

11. Covalently connects segments of DNA. 11_____

12. Synthesizes short segments of RNA. 12_____

13. Resolves catenates of DNA. 13_____

Questions 14-18.

DIRECTIONS: Each group of questions below consists of five lettered headings followed by a list of numbered phrases or sentences. For each numbered phrase or sentence, select the one heading that is MOST closely related to it. One heading may be used once, more than once, or not at all.

A. Eukaryotic chromosome
B. Plasma membrane
C. Bacterial ribosome
D. Bacterial plasmid pBR322
E. Microtubule

14. Many of its proteins are involved in hydrophobic interactions with phospholipids. 14____

15. Proteins are the only major kind of macromolecule present. 15____

16. Most of its proteins are rich in lysine or arginine. 16____

17. A single copy of each of about 50 different protein molecules is present. 17____

18. A significant amount of uracil and no thymidine is present. 18____

19. When the outcome of an infection with a temperate bacteriophage (such as lambda) is stable lysogeny, which of the following virus genes is expressed in the host cell? 19____

A. Lysozyme gene
B. Capsid protein gene
C. Receptor
D. Represser
E. Antirepressor

20. Which of the following eukaryotic DNA control sequences does NOT need to be in a fixed location and is MOST responsible for high rates of transcription from particular genes? 20____

A. Enhancer sequence
B. Promoter sequence
C. TATA box
D. Polyadenylation sequence
E. Represser sequence

21. Which of the following is TRUE for both prokaryotic and eukaryotic gene expression? 21____

A. After transcription, a 3' poly A tail and a 5' cap are added to mRNA.
B. Translation of mRNA can begin before transcription is complete.
C. RNA polymerase may recognize a promoter region upstream from the gene.
D. mRNA is synthesized in the 3' to 5' direction.
E. The mRNA transcript is always colinear to the gene from which it was copied.

22. The few viable interspecies hybrids are usually sterile (e.g., the mule, obtained from crossing a horse with a donkey, or the dzo, obtained from crossing a cow with a yak). The MOST likely cause for this type of hybrid sterility is 22____

A. meiotic drive
B. lack of homologous pairing
C. lack of premeiotic chromosome duplication
D. nonhomologous crossing over
E. nonmaturation of sex organs

23. After a series of steps that include dehydration, phosphoryl transfer to ADP, and reduction by NADH, which of the following structures is formed in the glycolytic pathway under anaerobic conditions? 23____

A. 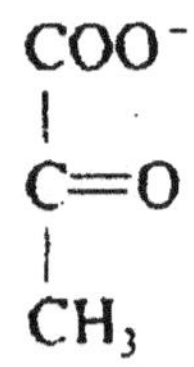

B. 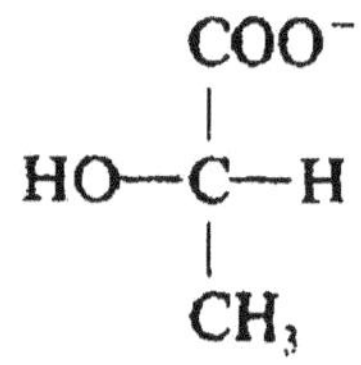

C. 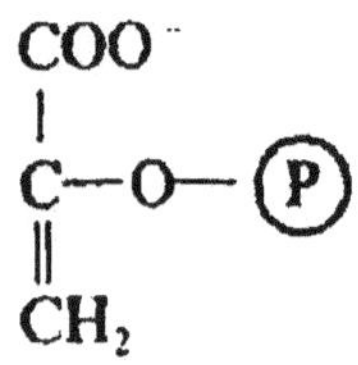

D. 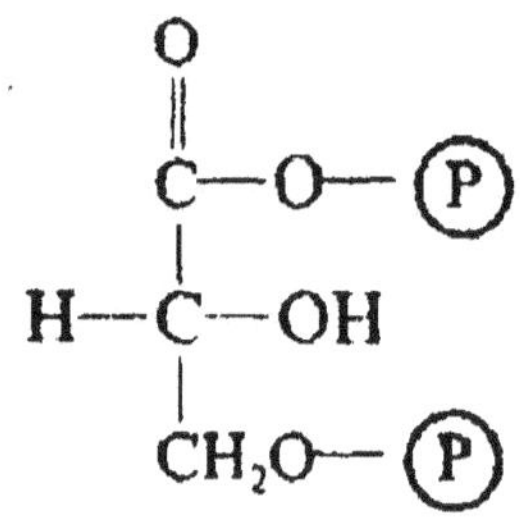

E. 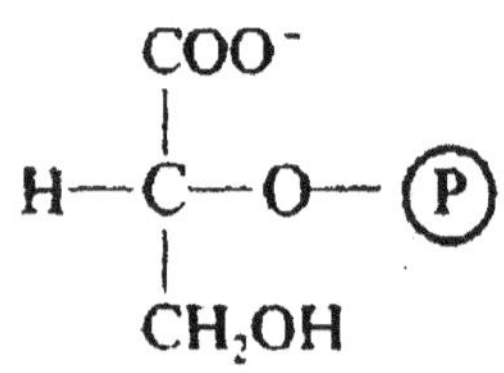

24. Substrate-level phosphorylation occurs in which of the following pairs of processes? 24____

A. Photosynthesis and glycolysis
B. Glycolysis and citric acid (Krebs) cycle
C. Photosynthesis and citric acid (Krebs) cycle
D. Citric acid (Krebs) cycle and coupled mitochondrial electron transport
E. Glycolysis and coupled mitochondrial electron transport

25. The addition of sialic acid to the carbohydrate moiety of a secretory glyco-protein is MOST likely to occur in the 25____

A. Golgi complex
B. lysosome
C. endoplasmic reticulum
D. coated vesicle
E. endosome

Questions 26-27.

DIRECTIONS: Questions 26 and 27 concern an experimental situation. First study the description of the situation. Then choose the one BEST answer to each question following it.

Regulatory enzymes are subject to both allosteric and covalent regulation. Proteases can digest these enzymes into separate catalytic and regulatory domains, revealing the spatial organization of the enzymes. In the following example, a regulatory enzyme is either phosphorylated with a protein kinase or briefly digested with a protease. Following treatment, the regulatory enzyme is assayed for activity in the presence or absence of an allosteric effector. The results of the experiment are as follows:

Treatment	Relative Activity Without Effector	With Effector
None	10	80
Kinase	80	120
Protease	80	80

26. Which of the following can be concluded about the effects of phosphorylation of the regulatory enzyme? 26____
It

A. produces an active conformation that is not influenced by the effector
B. produces an active conformation that can be further activated by the effector
C. changes conformation to increase basal activity without altering interaction with the effector
D. changes interaction of catalytic and regulatory domains to eliminate influence of the effector
E. leads to autoproteolysis of the enzyme

27. Which of the following statements explains how digestion with a protease causes activation of this enzyme? 27____
It removes a(n)

A. phosphorylation site in the catalytic domain
B. inhibitory regulatory domain
C. segment blocking the effector binding site
D. substrate binding site on the catalytic domain
E. activation site from the regulatory domain

Questions 28-30.

DIRECTIONS: Questions 28 through 30 concern an experimental situation. First study the description of the situation. Then choose the one BEST answer to each question following it.

The *E. coli* bacterial chromosome is circular. The unidirectional transfer of the chromosome from a donor Hfr strain to a recipient F^- strain occurs when the Hfr exists at different locations in the chromosome of the donor and mobilizes the donor chromosome in one of two possible directions, depending on the orientation of insertion of the Hfr into the donor chromosome. Consider the table of data below, which lists the observed frequency of appearance of wild-type recombinants for the four genetic markers given, using each of the three different Hfr donor strains.

Donor Strain	Marker Frequency (%) in F^--Recipient			
	Ilv^+	Lac^+	His^+	Arg^+
Hfr_1	80.0	30.0	5.0	0.03
Hfr_2	0.5	0.07	0.01	1.5
Hfr_3	0.05	32.0	5.0	0.1

28. The order of gene loci on the circular bacterial chromosome is 28____

A. *lac* → *ilv* → *his* → *arg*
B. *lac* → *his* → *arg* → *ilv*
C. *lac* → *his* → *ilv* → *arg*
D. *lac* → *arg* → *his* → *ilv*
E. *lac* → *arg* → *ilv* → *his*

29. The location and direction of transfer of Hfr_3 in the bacterial chromosome is between ______ in the direction of ______ . 29____

A. *his* and *arg* ; *arg*
B. *his* and *arg*; *his*
C. *ilv* and *lac*; *lac*
D. *ilv* and *lac* ; *ilv*
E. *arg* and *ilv*, *ilv*

30. The largest region of the chromosome that is mapped LEAST well lies between 30____

A. *arg* and *ilv*
B. Hfr_1 and *lac*
C. *his* and *arg*
D. *lac* and *his*
E. *ilv* and *lac*

31. Which of the following events is immediately induced in an early G_1 cell when it is fused with an S-phase cell, but not when it is fused with a G_2 cell? 31____

A. Cytokinesis
B. Mitosis
C. Chromosome condensation
D. DNA replication
E. Nuclear envelope disruption

32. When the concentration of KCl is raised from 0.015 molar to 0.15 molar, G-actin spontaneously polymerizes into which of the following structures? 32____
A(n)

A. helix
B. antiparallel beta-pleated sheet
C. parallel beta-pleated sheet
D. beta-turn
E. random coil

33. All of the following are usually associated with trans-posable elements (transposons) EXCEPT 33____

A. acquisition of resistance to antibiotics by bacteria
B. an enzyme that catalyzes insertion into new sites
C. inverted repeats
D. insertion into preexisting DNA by homologous recombination
E. probable presence in all organisms

34. In a double-stranded DNA molecule of random sequence, which of the following restriction enzymes will cut the molecule LEAST often? (In the sequence of bases for each recognition site, N = any base, P = either purine base, and Y = either pyrimidine base.) 34____

	Restriction Enzyme	Recognition Site
A.	*Alu*I	AGCT
B.	*Bgl*I	GCCNNNNNGGC
C.	*Sfi*I	GGCCNNNNNGGCC
D.	*BspM*I	ACCTC
E.	*Hind*II	GTYPAC

Questions 35-37.

DIRECTIONS: Questions 35 through 37 are to be answered on the basis of the following information and diagrams.

Salivary glands were incubated briefly with ^{3}H-leucine, washed, and then incubated with nonradioactive amino acids for varying times. The tissue was fixed, embedded, sectioned, and subjected to auto-radiography. Electron microscopy revealed a grain pattern, as seen in Figures X, Y, and Z below. (A silver grain is represented by γ .)

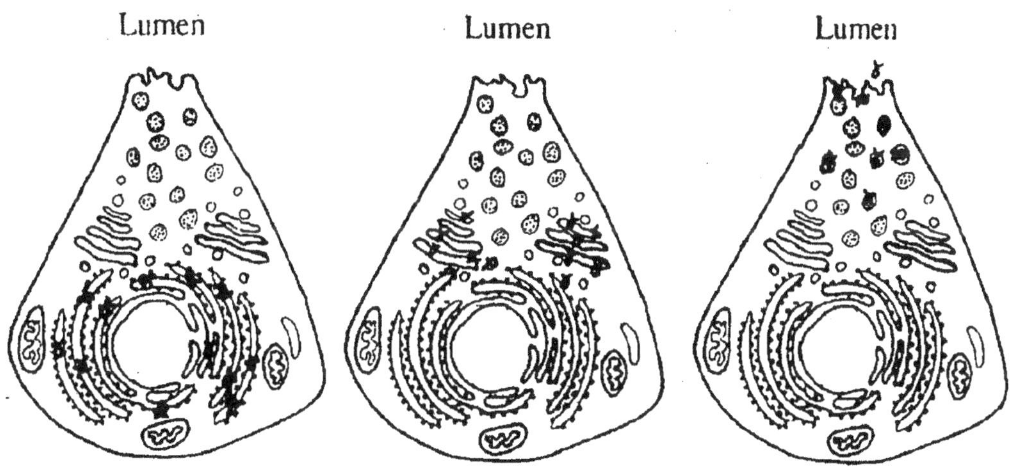

Figure X
4 min. after initial exposure

Figure Y
25 min. after initial exposure

Figure Z
100 min. after initial exposure

35. This study illustrates the synthesis of 35____

A. proteins
B. carbohydrates
C. lipids
D. DNA
E. RNA

36. The aim of this experiment is to determine the 36____

A. identity of macromolecules within secretory vesicles
B. function of the smooth endoplasmic reticulum
C. path of movement of secreted molecules from initial synthesis to eventual secretion
D. stimulus for secretion of the product into the lumen
E. function of the secreted molecules while they move through the cell

37. The strategy used in this experiment is referred to as 37____

A. pulse-chase analysis
B. Southern blot
C. immunocytochemical localization
D. *in situ* hybridization
E. restriction mapping

38. A 0.05-percent solution of a pure protein has an absorbance of 0.34 at 280 nanometers in a cuvette with a 1-centimeter path length. 38____
Which of the following is CLOSEST to the concentration of the same protein in a solution with an absorbance of 0.75 at 280 nanometers in a cuvette with a 1-centimeter path length?
_______ $mg \cdot mL^{-1}$

A. 0.11 B. 0.91 C. 1.1 D. 9.1 E. 11

39. All of the following are integral components of the mammalian inner mitochondrial membrane EXCEPT 39____

A. succinate dehydrogenase
B. ATP synthase
C. NADH dehydrogenase
D. catalase
E. cytochrome a_3

40. Chemicals that inhibit DNA synthesis can be used to treat cancer in humans because 40____

A. noncancerous cells do not synthesize DNA
B. noncancerous cells are resistant to the chemicals
C. cancer is caused by alterations in DNA
D. cancerous cells revert to the normal state when DNA synthesis is inhibited
E. cancerous cells generally divide more frequently than noncancerous cells

41. Into which two compartments are protons (H^+) pumped during respiration and photosynthesis, respectively? The 41____

A. intermembrane space of a mitochondrion and the inter-membrane space of a chloroplast
B. intermembrane space of a mitochondrion and the thylakoid lumen of a chloroplast
C. intermembrane space of a mitochondrion and the stroma of a chloroplast
D. matrix of a mitochondrion and the thylakoid lumen of a chloroplast
E. matrix of a mitochondrion and the stroma of a chloroplast

42. The maximum useful work that can be obtained from a chemical reaction operating in a perfectly reversible manner at constant temperature and pressure is termed 42____

A. work function
B. entropy
C. enthalpy
D. free energy
E. internal energy

43. Which of the following pairs of molecules exhibits sp^3 hybridization of their bonding orbitals? 43____

A. Ethylene and propylene
B. Acetylene and carbon monoxide
C. Acetylene and ethylene
D. Methane and methanol
E. Propylene and cyclopropane

44. Which of the following types of enzyme inhibitors changes the apparent K_M, while having no effect on the V_{max}? 44____

A. Irreversible
B. Noncompetitive
C. Competitive
D. Uncompetitive
E. Suicide

KEY (CORRECT ANSWERS)

1. A	11. C	21. C	31. D	41. B
2. D	12. E	22. B	32. A	42. D
3. C	13. D	23. B	33. D	43. D
4. B	14. B	24. B	34. C	44. C
5. C	15. E	25. A	35. A	
6. D	16. A	26. B	36. C	
7. D	17. C	27. B	37. A	
8. E	18. C	28. B	38. C	
9. D	19. D	29. C	39. D	
10. A	20. A	30. C	40. E	

EXAMINATION SECTION
TEST 1

DIRECTIONS: Each question or incomplete statement is followed by several suggested answers or completions. Select the one that BEST answers the question or completes the statement. *PRINT THE LETTER OF THE CORRECT ANSWER IN THE SPACE AT THE RIGHT.*

1. A purulent infection of a meibomian gland of the eyelid is termed 1.____

   A. meibomianitis
   B. blephritis
   C. external hordeolum
   D. internal hordeolum

2. A woman comes in with flat yellow lesions of the lids, composed of lipids. Lesions arched in wing-shaped fashion in the region of the nasal canthi are termed 2.____

   A. dermoid
   B. chalazion
   C. xanthelasma
   D. hemangiomas

3. A tumor of the eyelids which has an elevated epithelial nodule with an umbilicated center and the etiology of a low virulence virus is called a 3.____

   A. hemangioma
   B. lymphangioma
   C. sebaceous cyst
   D. molluscum contagiosum

4. What is the MOST common organism responsible for approximately two-thirds of all observed ocular inflammations and infections? 4.____

   A. Pseudomonas aeruginosa
   B. Staphylococcus aureus
   C. Staphylococcus epidermidis
   D. Hemophilus influenzae

5. A granulomatous inflammation of a meibomian gland resulting from resolution of an internal hordeolum appearing as a non-tender and well-circumscribed lump on the lid is called a 5.____

   A. chalazion
   B. xanthelasma
   C. papilloma
   D. chloasma

6. Slightly elevated lesions with pearly margins and an ulcerated center, usually associated with telangiectasias, describes a _______ carcinoma. 6.____

   A. squamous cell
   B. basal cell
   C. lymphosarcoma
   D. ulcerative blephritis

7. A 27 year-old female patient is present with bilateral and symmetrical dry, hyperemic, wrinkled, and irritated lids. She provides a history of using a new skin product recently. Her chief complaint is of pruritis. What is the MOST likely diagnosis? 7.____

   A. Seborrheic blephritis
   B. Contact dermatitis of lids
   C. Ulcerative blephritis
   D. None of the above

8. A 62 year-old comes to the office with complaints of ocular burning and irritation, especially in the morning. On examination, you notice sheathing debris build-up at the base of the cilia. 8.____
What is the MOST likely diagnosis?

A. Keratitis sicca
B. Contact dermatitis
C. Demodex folliculorum
D. Allergy of the lids

9. All of the following are true regarding chronic infantile dacrocystitis EXCEPT: 9.____

A. It always requires surgical intervention
B. Daily massage of the lacrimal sac is indicated
C. Probing should be delayed until 6 months of age
D. It results from failure of canalization of the naso-lacrimal duct at birth

10. All of the following are true regarding treatment of acute dacryocystitis EXCEPT: 10.____

A. Initiate lacrimal dilation and irrigation after resolution
B. Use topical antibiotic drops or ointment
C. No systemic therapy is indicated
D. Use a warm compress

11. Dacroadenitis is NOT caused by 11.____

A. degenerative enlargement
B. bacterial inflammation
C. systemic viral inflammation
D. expired eye drops

12. A 28 year-old female comes to your office with unilateral tearing of six months duration. Her eyes are white except for mucous regurgitation from the lacrimal sac. 12.____
The MOST likely diagnosis is

A. acute dacryocystitis
B. keratoconjunctivitis sicca
C. canaliculitis
D. chronic dacryocystitis

13. An 18 year-old male patient is diagnosed as having conjunctivitis due to chlamydia specie. 13.____
The drug of choice is oral

A. ampicillin
B. tetracycline
C. streptomycin
D. prednisone

14. A patient comes in with a bright red, sharply delineated area on the bulbar conjunctiva of one eye. It is surrounded by normal conjunctiva. 14.____
The MOST likely diagnosis is

A. pink eye
B. naevus flammeus
C. sub-conjunctival hemorrhage
D. episcleritis

15. Proliferation of hyaline and elastic tissue that replaces Bowman's membrane of the cornea is commonly seen in patients living in warm climates with frequent exposure to dusty environments. 15.____
The MOST likely diagnosis is

A. pannus
B. pterygium
C. hemangioma
D. pinguecula

16. A 9 year-old boy is brought to your office complaining of itching in both eyes. His superior palpabral conjunctivae contain large cobblestone-like papillae and a milky, mucoid discharge. 16.____
The MOST likely diagnosis is

A. trachoma
B. palpabral vernal conjunctivitis
C. limbal vernal conjunctivitis
D. all of the above

17. An 8 year-old boy is struck in the eye by a tree branch while playing. An area of conjunctival edema and hyper-emia has developed. The lesion stains with sodium fluorescein but does not reveal bare sclera. 17.____
Your diagnosis is

A. conjunctival abrasion
B. conjunctival foreign body
C. subconjunctival hemorrhage
D. none of the above

18. A 22 year-old female patient comes to your office with itchy eyes, lid edema, and chemosis with a mucous discharge. She recently got a pet cat. 18.____
What is the MOST likely diagnosis?

A. Contact dermatitis
B. Pink eye
C. Erythema nodosum
D. Allergic blepharcoconjunctivitis

19. What is the APPROPRIATE treatment for the patient mentioned in the previous question? 19.____

A. Antihistamines and topical steroids
B. Mast cell stabilizers
C. Avoidance of the causative agent
D. All of the above

20. ______ ulcers are known for their creeping, which destroys corneal tissue and causes perforation. 20.____

A. Streptococcal
B. Marginal
C. Dendritic
D. None of the above

21. ______ are signs of an aging cornea. 21.____

A. Wart-like excrescences over the descemets membrane
B. Hassall Henle bodies

C. Guttata
D. All of the above

22. Which of the following is TRUE regarding arcus senilis? 22.____

A. A narrow white band of lipid infiltration is separated from the limbus by a clear zone
B. It occurs in almost everyone by the age of 80
C. It may or may not be associated with increased blood cholesterol levels
D. All of the above

23. Epidemic keratoconjunctivitis is 23.____

A. not an infectious condition
B. caused by the adenovirus that causes the common cold
C. not associated with fever
D. not associated with photophobia

24. Which of the following is TRUE regarding orbital cellulitis? 24.____

A. It causes the eyelids to become swollen shut.
B. It is accompanied by chemosis.
C. It is accompanied by fever and exopthalmos.
D. All of the above

25. Complications of orbital cellulitis are 25.____

A. its spread to the cavernous sinus
B. thrombosis and death
C. both of the above
D. none of the above

KEY (CORRECT ANSWERS)

1. D
2. C
3. D
4. B
5. A

6. B
7. B
8. C
9. A
10. C

11. D
12. D
13. B
14. C
15. B

16. B
17. A
18. D
19. D
20. A

21. D
22. D
23. B
24. D
25. C

TEST 2

DIRECTIONS: Each question or incomplete statement is followed by several suggested answers or completions. Select the one that BEST answers the question or completes the statement. *PRINT THE LETTER OF THE CORRECT ANSWER IN THE SPACE AT THE RIGHT.*

1. A patient comes in with pimples on her eyelid margin, external to the eyelashes. Your diagnosis is styes due to infection. 1.____
The treatment should consist of

A. hot soaks B. local antibiotics
C. incision D. all of the above

2. Ptosis, which is a drooping lid that rests more than 2 mm below corneal margin, may be due to 2.____

A. congenital defects B. insomnia
C. ptyalism D. all of the above

3. First aid for chemical injuries to the eye includes 3.____

A. patching the eye
B. antibiotic eye drops
C. irrigation with water and normal saline
D. irrigation with an alkali solution

4. Exophthalmos is defined as an abnormal protrusion of the eyeball. 4.____
It may be the result of

A. thyroid disease in adult cases
B. orbital cellulitis in child cases
C. metastatic tumors
D. all of the above

5. When an immune reaction to mucus debris on soft contact lenses leads to development of large papillae under the eyelids. 5.____
The MOST common cause for rejection is

A. vernal conjunctivitis
B. giant papillary conjunctivitis
C. trachoma
D. inclusion conjunctivitis

6. What treatment is APPROPRIATE for giant papillary conjunctivitis that develops as a result of soft contact lens rejection? 6.____

A. Incision
B. Keep lenses especially clean
C. IV antibiotics
D. All of the above

7. The MOST common cause of conjunctivitis in newborns who acquire it passing through the birth canal is 7.____

A. chlamydia trachomatis
B. streptococcus
C. staphylococcus aureus
D. none of the above

8. Which of the following is TRUE regarding episcleritis? 8.____

A. It is a localized superficial inflammation of the episclera.
B. It adversely affects visual acuity.
C. Treatment with antihistamines or antibiotics has been prescribed.
D. All of the above

9. All of the following are true of scleritis EXCEPT that 9.____

A. juvenile rheumatoid arthritis is a common cause
B. it is painful
C. it often includes intraocular involvement
D. it is incurable

10. Blue sclera may be found in all of the following EXCEPT 10.____

A. scleral thinning
B. increased uveal pigmentation
C. in children as a normal finding
D. none of the above

11. All of the following are signs and symptoms of acute anterior uveitis EXCEPT 11.____

A. ciliary flush
B. dilated immobile pupils
C. pain
D. photophobia

12. Which of the following is TRUE regarding chronic anterior uveitis? 12.____

A. Patients have symptoms of reduced visual acuity.
B. Patients have redness of the eye.
C. It is never accompanied by any systemic disease.
D. It is always unilateral.

13. Which of the following are signs and symptoms of albinism? 13.____

A. Macular hypoplasia
B. Nystagmus
C. Prominent choroidal vasculature
D. All of the above

14. A patient comes in with eye problems. Upon examination, you find that one pupil exhibits a sluggish reaction to light and to near. The affected pupil stays larger than that of the other eye in bright light and smaller in dim light. 14.____
The MOST likely diagnosis is

A. pupillary block
B. adies tonic pupil
C. Argyll Robertson pupil
D. none of the above

15. Acquired hyperopia is USUALLY seen in which of the following conditions? 15.____

A. Diabetes
B. Orbital tumor
C. Macular cyst
D. All of the above

16. Following blunt trauma, a 27 year-old patient exhibits unilateral, enophthalmus, restricted elevation of the globe of the eye and intraorbital nerve hypoesthesia. The MOST likely diagnosis is 16.____

A. blow-out fracture
B. Grave's ophthalmos
C. traumatic rupture of the eyeball
D. none of the above

17. An 8 year-old patient sustained a penetrating injury to his upper eyelid and received no treatment. Two to three days later, he comes to the office with periorbital redness, edema, and localized tenderness. No ocular involvement is experienced. The MOST likely diagnosis is 17.____

A. orbital cellulitis
B. preseptal cellulitis
C. delayed allergic reaction
D. none of the above

18. Which of the following is TRUE of primary open angle glaucoma? 18.____

A. It is the most common form of glaucoma
B. It is a familial disorder
C. Both of the above
D. None of the above

19. In primary open angle glaucoma, ______ is the cause of obstruction to aqueous outflow. 19.____

A. trabecular meshwork
B. a ciliary body
C. trachoma
D. corneal endothelium

20. The ______ cataract is the MOST common congenital form of cataracts. 20.____

A. stellate
B. anterior axial embryonal
C. anterior polar or pyramidal
D. posterior polar

21. Which of the following conditions may lead to cataract formation? 21.____

A. Systemic steroid usage
B. Chronic anterior uveitis
C. Ocular contusion
D. All of the above

22. All of the following statements are true regarding a late rosette cataract EXCEPT that 22.____

A. it may develop in years following ocular contusion
B. late rosette cataract is permanent
C. late rosette cataract is reversible
D. it results in a petal-shaped opacity

23. Which of the following cataracts is NOT related to age? 23.____

A. Cupulliform B. Cuneiform
C. Pulvurulent D. Crystalline

24. Flame-shaped hemorrhages in the superficial retinal layers may be found in 24.____

A. diabetic retinopathy
B. hypertensive retinopathy
C. papilledema
D. all of the above

25. Roll's spots may be found in 25.____

A. diffuse choroidal sclerosis
B. leukemia
C. hypertensive retinopathy
D. syphilitic chorioretinitis

KEY (CORRECT ANSWERS)

1.	D	11.	B
2.	A	12.	A
3.	C	13.	D
4.	D	14.	B
5.	B	15.	D
6.	B	16.	A
7.	A	17.	B
8.	A	18.	C
9.	D	19.	A
10.	D	20.	B

21. D
22. C
23. C
24. D
25. B

EXAMINATION SECTION
TEST 1

DIRECTIONS: Each question or incomplete statement is followed by several suggested answers or completions. Select the one that BEST answers the question or completes the statement. *PRINT THE LETTER OF THE CORRECT ANSWER IN THE SPACE AT THE RIGHT.*

1. What is the MOST common retinal finding in patients suffering from acquired immune deficiency syndrome? 1.____

   A. Cotton wool patches
   B. Hard exudates
   C. Neovasculization
   D. Flame hemorrhages

2. Which of the following is consistent with optic atrophy? 2.____

   A. Reduced visual acuity
   B. Optic disc pallor
   C. Afferent pupillary defect
   D. All of the above

3. Papillitis and papilledema appear ophthalmoscopically similar. What evaluation of optic nerve function is ESSENTIAL to differentiate between the two? 3.____

   A. Visual acuity measurement
   B. Color vision assessment
   C. Visual field analysis
   D. All of the above

4. A 32 year-old male comes in complaining of monocular visual loss lasting 15 minutes followed by ipsilateral headache. Upon examination, the patient appears to be in good physical health. Fundoscopic examination and visual field analysis are all normal. What is the MOST likely diagnosis? 4.____

   A. Ophthalmic migraine
   B. Ocular migraine
   C. Common migraine
   D. Migraine equivalent

5. Bell's palsy 5.____

   A. causes unilateral facial paralysis
   B. arises from paralysis of sympathetic nerve
   C. is always permanent
   D. involves III cranial nerve

6. A patient comes in exhibiting symptoms of ptosis, extropia, loss of accommodation, and a dilated, non-reactive pupil. You suspect total oculomotor ophthalmoplegia. The MOST common cause for it is 6.____

   A. trauma
   B. carotid aneurysm
   C. diabetes
   D. all of the above

7. Which of the following clinical instruments is used to perform corneal curvature measurements? 7.____

A. Ophthalmometer
B. Video photokeratoscope
C. Genioscope
D. None of the above

8. Which instrument is used to measure corneal thickness? 8.____

A. Direct ophthalmoscope
B. Slit lamp
C. Optical pachymeter
D. Genioscope

9. What is the purpose of binocular balancing? 9.____

A. To balance the state of accommodation
B. To balance visual acuity
C. To check for astigmatism
D. None of the above

10. Which of the following clinical techniques is used in obtaining binocular balance? 10.____

A. Dichrome test
B. Prism dissociation
C. Keratoplasty
D. All of the above

11. Tinted lenses are useful in all of the following conditions EXCEPT 11.____

A. elimination of reflected glare
B. reduction of the intensity of UV radiation entering the eye
C. cosmetic improvement
D. reduction of the intensity of infrared radiation entering the eye

12. Which of the following conditions is NOT considered a leading cause of blindness? 12.____

A. Diabetic retinopathy
B. Trauma
C. Age-related maculopathy
D. Glaucoma

13. The condition that occurs when parallel rays of light are focused behind the retina is called 13.____

A. myopia
B. presbyopia
C. hyperopia
D. emmetropia

14. The causes of paralytic strabismus do NOT include 14.____

A. eye muscle weakness from thyroid disease
B. orbital floor fractures
C. glaucoma
D. traumatic contusions

15. Aphakic patients with ______ benefit from extended wear contact lenses. 15.____

A. senility
B. arthritis
C. unsteady hands
D. all of the above

16. The condition in which two ocular images are different in size and/or shape is called 16.____

A. aniseikonia
B. amblyopia
C. myopia
D. none of the above

17. All of the following conditions may be treated effectively with optical aids EXCEPT 17.____

A. aphakia
B. keratoconus
C. advanced glaucoma
D. myopia

18. Amblyopia is often found in association with which of the following? 18.____

A. Antimetropia
B. Congenital cataracts
C. Esotropia
D. All of the above

19. A patient has a paresis of the superior rectus of the left eye. 19.____
In order for the patient to maintain orthotropia, his head posture would BEST be

A. face up and to the right, head tilted to the right
B. face down and to the right, head tilted to the right
C. face down and to the left, head tilted to the left
D. face up and to the left, head tilted to the left

20. What is the treatment for amblyopia? 20.____

A. Patching non-amblyopic eye
B. Patching the amblyopic eye
C. Rotating gratings
D. All of the above

21. A prominent epicanthal fold can lead to the false diagnosis of 21.____

A. hypotropia
B. esotropia
C. exotropia
D. hypermetropia

22. When the angle of squint remains fairly constant in all fields of gaze, the squint is said to be 22.____

A. paralytic
B. concomitant
C. anomalous
D. none of the above

23. A nystagmus present only when the patient gazes in the direction of the fast component is termed _______ degree. 23.____

A. first
B. second
C. third
D. fourth

24. The CA/C ratio describes the 24.____

A. amount of accommodation elicited by convergence
B. amount of convergence elicited by accommodation
C. degree of myopia
D. none of the above

25. The AC/A ratio 25.____

A. describes the ratio of convergence in prism diaptors driven by accommodation to the accommodation in diap-ters
B. tends to be high in uncorrected myopes
C. both of the above
D. neither of the above

KEY (CORRECT ANSWERS)

1. A
2. D
3. D
4. B
5. A
6. D
7. B
8. C
9. A
10. B
11. A
12. B
13. C
14. C
15. D
16. A
17. C
18. D
19. A
20. D
21. B
22. B
23. A
24. A
25. C

TEST 2

DIRECTIONS: Each question or incomplete statement is followed by several suggested answers or completions. Select the one that BEST answers the question or completes the statement. *PRINT THE LETTER OF THE CORRECT ANSWER IN THE SPACE AT THE RIGHT.*

1. Conditions that produce retinal hypoxia may result in neovasculization. Which of the following conditions may lead to the development of neovasculization? 1.____

   A. Sickle cell retinopathy B. Retinal vein occlusion
   C. Diabetic retinopathy D. All of the above

2. What is the GREATEST contraindication to contact lens wear? 2.____

   A. Conjunctivitis
   B. Astigmatism greater than 2.50D
   C. Lack of motivation
   D. All of the above

3. The amount of oxygen retained beneath the contact lens with each blink is dependent upon which of the following factors? 3.____

   A. The amount of tears exchanged with each blink
   B. The frequency of blinking
   C. The volume of the tear reservoir behind the contact lens
   D. All of the above

4. All of the following favor protein deposit build-up on soft contact lenses EXCEPT 4.____

   A. incomplete blinking
   B. thermal disinfection
   C. altered tear composition
   D. chemical disinfection

5. Oxygen transmission through a contact lens is inversely related to the 5.____

   A. lens thickness
   B. water content of the lens material
   C. diameter of the lens
   D. all of the above

6. Oxygen transmission through a lens is directly proportional to the 6.____

   A. lens thickness
   B. water content of the lens material
   C. diameter of the lens
   D. all of the above

7. Which of the following is a TRUE statement regarding disposable lenses? They are 7.____

   A. not available in high astigmatic corrections
   B. available in a wide range of myopic and hyperopic corrections

C. very comfortable and convenient
D. all of the above

8. _______ lenses are associated with acanthamoeba infection. 8._____

A. Daily soft wear
B. Disposable
C. Extended wear
D. Rigid hard

9. What are the causes of acanthamoeba keratitis infection associated with contact lens use? 9._____

A. Disinfecting and storage solutions
B. Absence of sterile saline solutions
C. Saline solutions made with salt tablets and non-sterile distilled water
D. All of the above

10. The acanthamoeba organism CANNOT 10._____

A. penetrate corneal epithelium
B. contaminate lens care systems
C. adhere to contact lens
D. none of the above

11. Children with cerebral palsy exhibit an unusually high incidence of 11._____

A. strabismus
B. refractive errors
C. accomodative disorders
D. all of the above

12. Which condition has a HIGH incidence in Down's syndrome patients? 12._____

I. Cataracts
II. Strabismus
III. Ecotropia
IV. Antimetropia

The CORRECT answer is:

A. I *only*
B. III *only*
C. I, II
D. III, IV

13. Which of the following vision problems are associated with complete achromatopsia? 13._____

A. Photophobia
B. Blurred vision
C. Myopia
D. Cataracts

14. Which instrument is used for the assessment of retinal function in patients with cataracts? 14._____

A. Brightness acuity tester
B. Potential acuity meter
C. Vistech contrast sensitivity test
D. Pelli-Robson contrast sensitivity test

15. What are the common conditions in older people that lead to exaggerated disability glare? 15._____

A. Cataracts
B. Nuclear sclerosis
C. Corneal clouding
D. All of the above

16. In dealing with geriatric patients, you should 16.____

A. only answer questions from the patient's family
B. speak loudly
C. have extra patience and understanding
D. not tell the patient your diagnosis

17. What are the signs and symptoms of age-related macular degeneration? 17.____

A. Straight lines appear distorted
B. Peripheral vision remains good
C. Severe visual acuity loss
D. All of the above

18. The MOST commonly encountered color defect is 18.____

A. protanomaly
B. deuteranomaly
C. protanopia
D. tritanopia

19. Which of the following is normally observed in a rod monochromat? 19.____

A. Poor central acuity
B. Absence of color vision
C. Photophobia
D. All of the above

20. Doctors of optometry play an important role in the field of industrial/occupational vision by prescribing protective lenses. 20.____
What are common risk factors to the eye?

A. Excessive radiation and use of lasers
B. Inadequate lighting
C. Excessive moisture
D. All of the above

21. A(n) ______ epithelium is involved in the production of aqueous humor. 21.____

A. Retinal pigment
B. Unpigmented ciliary
C. Pigmented ciliary
D. None of the above

22. Which of the following is in the choroid layer? 22.____

A. Blood vessel vascular layer
B. Suprachoroid
C. Choriocapilaris
D. All of the above

23. What is the quantity of aqueous humor, in milliliters, normally contained in the anterior chamber? 23.____

A. 0.025
B. 235
C. 0.003
D. 0.25

24. Regarding the protein content of the lens, protein contributes ______% of the total weight of the lens. 24.____

A. 60
B. 10
C. 33
D. 100

25. The central retinal artery is a branch of the ______ artery. 25.____

A. ophthalmic
B. posterior ciliary
C. external carotid
D. none of the above

26. The nasolacrimal duct empties directly into the ______ meatus. 26.____

A. superior
B. middle
C. inferior
D. none of the above

27. What is the yoke muscle of the left lateral rectus? 27.____

A. Right medial rectus
B. Left medial rectus
C. Right lateral rectus
D. Right superior oblique

28. Which of the following features is NOT associated with Homer's syndrome? 28.____

A. Ptosis
B. Miosis
C. Anhidrosis
D. Sclerosis

29. The conjunctiva is NORMALLY covered by 29.____

A. epidermis
B. avascular membrane
C. mucous membrane
D. none of the above

30. Posterior conjunctiva arteries branch from the 30.____

A. major arterial circle of the iris
B. recurrent branches of the long posterior ciliary arteries
C. minor arterial circle of the iris
D. perforating branches of the palpebral arcades

KEY (CORRECT ANSWERS)

1. D
2. C
3. D
4. D
5. A

6. B
7. D
8. A
9. C
10. D

11. D
12. C
13. A
14. B
15. D

16. C
17. D
18. B
19. D
20. A

21. B
22. D
23. D
24. C
25. A

26. C
27. A
28. D
29. C
30. D

EXAMINATION SECTION
TEST 1

DIRECTIONS: Each question or incomplete statement is followed by several suggested answers or completions. Select the one that BEST answers the question or completes the statement. *PRINT THE LETTER OF THE CORRECT ANSWER IN THE SPACE AT THE RIGHT.*

1. The interior structures of the eye are studied with a 1.____

   A. tonometer
   B. ophthalmoscope
   C. gonioscope
   D. retinoscope
   E. orthorator

2. The organ MOST prone to occupational injuries is the 2.____

   A. eye
   B. ear
   C. skin
   D. lungs
   E. kidneys

3. Stereoscopic vision refers to 3.____

   A. the size of the visual field
   B. depth perception
   C. color perception
   D. image perception
   E. vision with two eyes

4. A perimeter is used to study 4.____

   A. depth perception
   B. near point abnormalities
   C. limit of the fields of vision
   D. monocular vision
   E. nocturnal acuity

5. The condition where the eyeball is too short from front to back is called 5.____

   A. nearsightedness
   B. poor depth perception
   C. night blindness
   D. farsightedness
   E. astigmatism

6. The unit of measure of the light-bending power of the lens is the 6.____

   A. angstrom
   B. micron
   C. index of refraction
   D. parsec
   E. diopter

7. Conjunctivitis is a(n) 7.____

   A. inflammation of the mucous membrane
   B. inflammation of the interior eye
   C. inflammation of the lacrimal gland
   D. inflammation of the tarsal gland
   E. cold sore

8. Early treatment of cold sores is necessary to prevent damage to the 8.____

A. conjunctiva
B. lacrimal gland
C. tarsal glands
D. retina
E. cornea

9. When the aqueous humor fails to drain properly, the ______ may be damaged. 9.____

A. retina
B. cornea
C. sclera
D. lens
E. optic nerve

10. The part of the eye MOST subject to attack is the 10.____

A. lens
B. cornea
C. iris
D. sclera
E. retina

11. The MOST prevalent form of occupational nystagmus is seen in 11.____

A. truck or long distance drivers
B. electronic factory workers
C. welders
D. miners
E. farmers

12. Displacement of the eyeball without rupture of the nerve is allowed by the 12.____

A. elasticity of the optic nerve
B. layers of the conjunctiva
C. length of the optic nerve
D. position of the optic nerve
E. bony ridge of the skull

13. The MOST common complication associated with industrial eye injuries is 13.____

A. dyslexia
B. blurred vision
C. infection
D. ambliopia
E. stagmus

14. A dark adapted eye will be LEAST affected by ______ light. 14.____

A. white
B. red
C. blue
D. green
E. yellow

15. Alkaline substances cause MORE severe eye damage than acidic chemicals because 15.____

A. alkaline substances continue to damage eye tissue as long as they remain on the eye
B. acids become dissolved by tears and weaken
C. alkaline substances are more highly ionic than acidic chemicals
D. there is no known neutralizing substance for alkaline chemicals
E. alkaline substances do not trigger a pain response and remain on the surface longer

16. Damage to cells of the lens due to irradiation burns may not be apparent for some time after insult because 16.____

A. the cells regenerate so quickly
B. there are few nerve endings
C. of the low level of metabolic activity
D. of the tearing mechanism
E. of not being well supplied with blood

17. If a concentrated caustic splashes in the eyes, the victim should 17.____

A. irrigate with a neutralizing solution
B. irrigate with boric acid solution
C. irrigate with mineral oil
D. irrigate with water
E. avoid self-help and report to the medical department

18. The test distance for near vision is 18.____

A. 56 cm
B. 20 feet
C. 6 inches
D. 2 feet
E. 14 inches

19. The eyelids contain tiny tarsal glands that lubricate the surface of the eyeball and eyelids with 19.____

A. mucus
B. water
C. oil
D. salt water
E. alkaline solution

20. The eye defect that can be corrected with concave lenses is 20.____

A. astigmatism
B. hyperopia
C. presbyopia
D. ambliopia
E. myopia

21. The visual screening program MUST include a test for 21.____

A. glaucoma
B. color perception
C. field of vision
D. visual acuity
E. depth perception

22. The white of the eye is called the 22.____

A. aqueous humor
B. choroid
C. vitreous humor
D. sclera
E. conjunctiva

23. A medical eye specialist is a(n) 23.____

A. ophthalmologist
B. retinologist
C. optician
D. optometrist
E. all of the above

24. The instrument used by the examiner to disclose any refractive aberration of the eye is the 24.____

A. ophthalmoscope
B. orthorator
C. retinoscope
D. corneal microscope
E. tonometer

25. An irregular curvature of the cornea results in 25.____

A. hyperopia
B. myopia
C. presbyopia
D. astigmatism
E. stereopsis

26. For the adaptation process to be complete, the eye should remain in total darkness for ______ minutes. 26.____

A. 3-5
B. 5-10
C. 10-15
D. 15-30
E. 30-60

27. An eye that becomes scratchy and red and has a discharge is *usually* suffering from 27.____

A. cold sores
B. trachcoma
C. glaucoma
D. conjunctivitis
E. eyestrain

28. The *leading* cause of blindness is 28.____

A. glaucoma
B. cataracts
C. conjunctivitis
D. syphilis
E. ophthalmic cancer

29. Glaucoma may develop as a result of 29.____

A. aging
B. infection
C. tumor
D. congenital defect
E. all of the above
F.

30. Reading without eyestrain is BEST accomplished by holding the paper or book ______ inches away. 30.____

A. 4-6
B. 6-10
C. 10-15
D. 16-18
E. more than 18

31. An object delivering a blow to the eye seals the rim of the bony orbit on impact, exerting hydraulic pressure. This type of blow may cause contusions of all the following EXCEPT the 31.____

A. iris
B. lens
C. cornea
D. retina
E. optic nerve

32. The CHIEF function of the teary blink is to 32.____

A. lubricate the surfaces of the eyeball and eyelids
B. wash foreign bodies from the corneal and conjunctival surfaces
C. clean the lens
D. fight bacteria
E. dissolve mildly toxic liquids

33. A person lacking *stereopsis* would have difficulty 33.____

A. focusing on distant objects
B. focusing on near objects
C. seeing at night
D. judging distance
E. identifying color

34. The increase of fluid pressure within the eye results in a condition called 34.____

A. conjunctivitis
B. glaucoma
C. astigmatism
D. hyperopia
E. myopia

35. Sunglasses may be worn indoors 35.____

A. under strong fluorescent lighting
B. under strong incandescent lighting
C. if the worker feels more comfortable wearing them
D. to dark-condition the eyes of workers who drive at night
E. sunglasses should never be worn indoors

36. The energy from infrared radiations is absorbed by the 36.____

A. aqueous humor
B. iris and pupil
C. cornea
D. mucous membrane
E. lens and retina

37. All of the following are advantages of plastic over glass lenses EXCEPT that they 37.____

A. have a higher resistance to breakage
B. have more favorable resistance to small objects moving at high rates of speed
C. have more abrasion resistance
D. take longer to fog
E. have greater resistance to hot materials

38. Diplopia is a condition that results in 38.____

A. double vision
B. poor depth perception
C. blurred vision
D. night blindness
E. involuntary eye movement

39. To provide for fine focusing of the incoming light beam, the lens shape is altered by the 39.____

A. ciliary body
B. choroid
C. iris
D. cornea
E. sclera

40. The reflex that will ALWAYS alert the worker that he has a foreign body in his eye is 40.____

A. pain
B. blinking
C. tearing
D. blurring of vision
E. none of the above

41. The bending of the parallel rays coming from an illuminated object to converge to a focus on the retina is done by the 41.____

I. cornea
II. lens
III. optic nerve
IV. pupil
V. iris

The CORRECT answer is:

A. I, II
B. I, III
C. I, IV, V
D. II, III
E. II, IV, V

42. The BEST clue to distance is provided by 42.____

A. accommodation
B. convergence
C. depth perception
D. movement parallax
E. divergence

43. Treatment for glaucoma may involve 43.____

A. surgery
B. corrective lenses
C. eye exercise
D. eye patches
E. transplant

44. Involuntary movement of the eyeballs occurs among workers who 44.____

A. subject their eyes to abnormal and unaccustomed movement
B. have exposure to glare
C. work, in low light environments
D. perform close work
E. work in high movement environments

45. A person's night vision will be more acute in the peripheral field than in the center of the field of vision because 45.____

A. less light is focused on the center of the retina
B. there are more cones on the periphery of the retina
C. there are almost no rods at the folvea
D. the area around the folvea is usually damaged from overexposure
E. light reaching the center of the retina must pass through the thickest portion of the lens

46. The toxic nature of certain metallic elements like ______ will cause destruction of the eye. 46.____

A. iron
B. aluminum
C. silver
D. copper
E. gold

47. Which of the following are NOT recommended for use in industry where eye protection is mandatory? 47.____
    I. Contact lenses
    II. Sunglasses
    III. Plastic lens glasses
    IV. Phototropic lens glasses
    V. Impact-resistant prescription glasses
    The CORRECT answer is:
    A. I, II
    B. I, II, III, IV
    C. I, II, IV
    D. I, II, IV, V
    E. all of the above

48. The front of the eyeball is protected by a smooth, transparent layer of tissue called the 48.____
    A. lens
    B. cornea
    C. iris
    D. sclera
    E. conjunctiva

49. Scattering of light within the eye is MINIMIZED by the 49.____
    A. pupil
    B. vitreous humor
    C. iris
    D. choroid
    E. ciliary body

50. The end result of a chemical burn is *usually* a scar on the 50.____
    A. lens
    B. iris
    C. sclera
    D. cornea
    E. eyelid

KEY (CORRECT ANSWERS)

1. B	11. D	21. D	31. C	41. A
2. A	12. C	22. D	32. B	42. C
3. B	13. C	23. A	33. D	43. A
4. C	14. B	24. C	34. B	44. A
5. D	15. A	25. D	35. E	45. C
6. E	16. C	26. E	36. E	46. D
7. A	17. D	27. D	37. C	47. D
8. E	18. E	28. A	38. A	48. E
9. E	19. C	29. E	39. A	49. D
10. B	20. E	30. D	40. E	50. D

EXAMINATION SECTION
TEST 1

DIRECTIONS: Each question or incomplete statement is followed by several suggested answers or completions. Select the one that BEST answers the question or completes the statement. *PRINT THE LETTER OF THE CORRECT ANSWER IN THE SPACE AT THE RIGHT.*

1. The instrument used to measure the pressures within the eyeball is a(n) 1.____

   A. gonioscope
   B. orthorator
   C. ophthalmoscope
   D. tonometer
   E. retinoscope

2. Protection of the eyes takes priority in any occupational safety and health program because 2.____

   A. the eye is prone to injury
   B. the eye is sensitive to more hazards
   C. the eye has no natural defenses
   D. injury to the eye affects other parts of the body
   E. the eye has fewer healing properties

3. The image on the right retina is 3.____

   A. the other half of the left retina's image
   B. a mirror image of the left retina's image
   C. more detailed than the left retina's image
   D. a slightly different image than the left retina's image
   E. an exact duplicate of the left retina's image

4. The instrument used to study the structure in the anterior part of the eye with high magnification is the 4.____

   A. orthorator
   B. corneal microscope
   C. window microscope
   D. retinoscope
   E. slit lamp microscope

5. The condition where the image of an object 20 feet away falls somewhere in front of the retina is called 5.____

   A. nearsightedness
   B. poor depth perception
   C. night blindness
   D. farsightedness
   E. astigmatism

6. The size of the pupil is changed through the action of the 6.____

   A. lens
   B. iris
   C. cornea
   D. optic nerve
   E. ciliary body

7. Conjunctivitis is *usually* caused by 7.____

   A. fungi
   B. bacteria
   C. a virus
   D. dust
   E. old age

8. Infection of the uveal tract damages the 8.____

I. retina
II. lens
III. cornea
IV. optic nerve
V. iris

The CORRECT answer is:

A. I, II, III
B. I, IV
C. II, III, IV
D. II, III, V
E. all of the above

9. Which of the following may be an indication of glaucoma? 9.____

A. Brightness of side vision
B. Appearance of colored rings and halos about bright objects
C. Double vision
D. Rapid shifts from acute to dull vision
E. Periodic episodes of an inability to focus on objects

10. Nystagmus is 10.____

A. excessive blinking
B. involuntary movement of the eyeballs
C. excessive tearing
D. inability to tear
E. night blindness

11. Serious irreversible injury can be caused by 11.____

A. displacement of the eyeball
B. foreign bodies affecting the conjunctiva
C. laceration of the lid
D. corneal laceration
E. contusion of the iris

12. The MOST common physical injury to the eye is 12.____

A. blows from blunt objects
B. retinal damage from sunlight
C. cut from sharp objects
D. foreign bodies
E. caustic chemicals

13. A cataract is an opaque spot that forms on the 13.____

A. retina
B. cornea
C. lens
D. iris
E. sclera

14. A plant vision conservation program would include all the following EXCEPT 14.____

A. a program to include 100% of the workers
B. attention to properly fitting eyewear
C. bonuses for workers demonstrating superior visual acuity

D. pre-employment eye examinations
E. posting warning signs such as: ALL PERSONNEL AND VISITORS MUST WEAR PROPER EYEWEAR

15. The harmful effects of the visible and ultraviolet radiation seen in welding will develop _______ after exposure. 15.____

A. within 5 minutes
B. 30-60 minutes
C. 2 hours
D. 6 hours
E. 24 hours

16. Coating plastic goggles with a hydrophylic coating prevents 16.____

A. abrasion
B. fogging
C. breakage
D. melting
E. shattering

17. No blood vessels are present in the 17.____

A. retina
B. sclera
C. iris
D. cornea
E. fovea

18. What distance do vision tests used in industry consider to be infinity? 18.____

A. 100 ft
B. 100 m
C. 20 ft
D. 10 m
E. 61 m

19. Additional problems in the control of ultraviolet light are associated with welding exceeding _______ amperes. 19.____

A. 10 B. 30 C. 5 D. 200 E. 1000

20. True loss of central vision is determined by 20.____

A. adding percentages of near and distant vision
B. dividing percentages of loss of distance vision by near vision
C. obtaining the mean of near and distant vision
D. adding the percentage of near and distant vision and subtracting the total from 100
E. doubling the near vision loss and adding the distant visual loss

21. The instrument used to study the angle of the chamber of the eye where the outflow drainage apparatus of the eye is found is a(n) 21.____

A. gonioscope
B. slit lamp microscope
C. ophthalmoscope
D. tonometer
E. retinoscope

22. Vision with two eyes is called 22.____

A. stereoscopic
B. panavision
C. binocular
D. dual
E. bi-ocular

23. About _______ percent of the population wears glasses. 23.____

A. 23 B. 40 C. 50 D. 60 E. 70

24. Farsightedness can be corrected with a ______ lens. 24.____

A. concave
B. convex
C. cylindrical
D. bi-concave
E. compound

25. Blurred vision, scarring and permanent damage to vision can be caused by 25.____

A. conjunctivitis
B. cold sores
C. glaucoma
D. trachcoma
E. cataracts

26. The MOST common form of glaucoma develops when 26.____

A. there is overproduction of vitreous humor
B. the lacrimal ducts are blocked
C. the diameter of the eye decreases
D. the aqueous humor fails to drain properly
E. the retina detaches

27. The "washers" of the eyes is (are) the 27.____

A. tarsal gland
B. eccrien glands
C. aqueous humor
D. lacrimal glands
E. apocrine glands

28. Which of the following would NOT have a direct effect on visual acuity? 28.____

A. Luminance
B. Position in the field
C. Duration
D. Contrast
E. Color

29. Kerato-conjunctivitis is a condition that may develop from a(n) 29.____

A. foreign object in the eye
B. chemical burn
C. loss of fluid from the eye
D. exposure to infrared light
E. exposure to excess ultraviolet light

30. If first aid measures are not taken in time, and a chemical penetrates the anterior chamber of the eye, the condition is called 30.____

A. irritis
B. acute keratitis
C. cataract
D. glaucoma
E. acute kerato-conjunctivitis

31. Visual acuity for distance should be recorded in the notation of 31.____

A. percent
B. point-type
C. fraction
D. decimal
E. inches

32. Light sensitive cells are contained in the 32.____

A. lens
B. choroid
C. optic nerve
D. cornea
E. retina

33. The eye defect that can be corrected with a cylindrical lens is 33.____

A. astigmatism
B. hyperopia
C. presbyopia
D. ambliopia
E. myopia

34. Monocular aphasia is considered a visual handicap. If present, it is assigned a value of ______ percent decrease in corrected central vision. 34.____

A. 5 B. 10 C. 20 D. 30 E. 50

35. The sclera 35.____

A. nourishes other tissues of the eye
B. protects and supports the eyeball
C. minimizes scattering of light
D. alters the shape of the lens
E. regulates the amount of light entering the eye

36. An ______ manufactures eyeglasses. 36.____

A. oculist
B. ophthalmologist
C. optician
D. ocular engineer
E. optometrist

37. A visual screening device that tests for acuity, depth, color,and vertical and lateral balance between the two eyes at various distances is a(n) 37.____

A. ophthalmoscope
B. gonioscope
C. Snellen Chart
D. perimeter
E. orthorator

38. The condition that results when the human lens lacks elasticity is 38.____

A. hyperopia
B. myopia
C. presbyopia
D. astigmatism
E. stereopsis

39. Optical cold sores *usually* affect the 39.____

A. mucous membrane
B. eyelid
C. anterior surface of the eyeball
D. interior of the eyelid
E. retina

40. Uveal inflammations are often associated with diseases of the 40.____

I. throat
II. joint
III. sinuses
IV. lung
V. intestinal tract

The CORRECT answer is:

A. I, II
B. I, II, III
C. I, II, IV
D. I, III, V
E. II, IV, V

41. Periodic eye examinations are essential to detect glaucoma because 41.____

A. the symptoms may be absent or go unnoticed
B. it affects other bodily systems
C. the symptoms are rarely eye-related
D. it is especially common among children
E. all of the above

42. The physician may diagnose night blindness when 42.____

A. there is weakness in the muscles of the iris
B. the patient complains of poor night vision
C. the ciliary muscles are weak
D. the eyeball is elongated
E. there is an irregularity of the cornea

43. Complaints of objects dancing before the eyes, headaches, dizziness and general fatigue are symptoms of 43.____

A. glaucoma
B. nystagmus
C. eyestrain
D. conjunctivitis
E. night blindness

44. The part of the eye that helps cushion the eyeball and tends to absorb impact is the 44.____

A. conjunctiva
B. sclera
C. uveal layer
D. aqueous humor
E. vitreous humor

45. The standard test for distance acuity is the 45.____

A. Snellen Chart
B. Jaeger Chart
C. Scale
D. Point Chart
E. Landolt's Broken-Ring Chart

46. Convergence, as part of stereoscopic acuity, is useful for distances up to 46.____

A. 20 meters
B. 1 meter or less
C. 100 meters
D. 5 meters
E. 1000 meters

47. According to American National Standard Z87, safety lenses must be *at least* ______ in thickness. 47.____

A. 1/16
B. 3 mm
C. 2 mm
D. 4 mm
E. 1/8 inch

48. Low-degree light damage to the lens is evidenced by 48.____

A. excessive tearing
B. dizziness
C. dimming of side vision
D. clouding of vision
E. appearance of bright spots

49. The eye protection equipment that offers MAXIMUM protection from flying particles is 49.____

A. flexible fitting goggles
B. chipping goggles
C. safety glasses
D. safety glasses with side shields
E. cushion fitting goggles

50. Illumination of the test chart for central visual acuity should be *at least* ______ lux. 50.____

A. 100 B. 50 C. 75 D. 25 E. 10

KEY (CORRECT ANSWERS)

1.	D	11.	E	21.	A	31.	C	41.	A
2.	E	12.	D	22.	C	32.	E	42.	B
3.	D	13.	C	23.	B	33.	A	43.	B
4.	E	14.	C	24.	B	34.	E	44.	A
5.	A	15.	D	25.	B	35.	B	45.	A
6.	B	16.	B	26.	D	36.	C	46.	A
7.	B	17.	D	27.	D	37.	E	47.	B
8.	A	18.	C	28.	E	38.	C	48.	D
9.	B	19.	B	29.	E	39.	C	49.	B
10.	B	20.	C	30.	A	40.	E	50.	B

EXAMINATION SECTION
TEST 1

DIRECTIONS: Each question or incomplete statement is followed by several suggested answers or completions. Select the one the BEST answers the question or completes the statement. *PRINT THE LETTER OF THE CORRECT ANSWER IN THE SPACE AT THE RIGHT.*

1. Which of the following symptoms is NOT consistent with normal pressure hydrocephalus? 1.____

   A. Gait disturbance
   B. Urinary incontinence
   C. Tachycardia
   D. Dementia

2. A 46-year-old woman, recently recovered from an upper respiratory infection, reports recent problems with vertigo, nausea, vomiting, and nystagmus. The symptoms have persisted for four days. The most likely disorder is 2.____

   A. vestibular neuritis
   B. cerebral aneurysm
   C. Guillain-Barre syndrome
   D. acoustic neuroma

3. An elderly man has fallen several times in the past few years, but has remained stable and never lost consciousness. He has recently developed increasing mental confusion associated with mild right hemiparesis, and a scan demonstrates compression in the left hemisphere. These findings are most consistent with 3.____

   A. hypertensive hemorrhage
   B. chronic subdural hematoma
   C. Alzheimer's disease
   D. epidural hematoma

4. Neuroreceptors are typically classified according to the 4.____

   A. frequency of their response to a stimulus
   B. type of stimulus they convert
   C. type of signal they produce
   D. speed with which they respond to a stimulus

5. Somatosensory input is received and interpreted by the brain's ______ lobe. 5.____

   A. frontal
   B. parietal
   C. temporal
   D. occipital

6. Treatments of Gullain-Barre syndrome include 6.____
   I. Early plasmapharesis
   II. Immunoglobulin infusion
   III. Orthotics
   IV. Tricyclic antidepressant medications

   A. I and II
   B. I, III and IV
   C. II only
   D. I, II, III and IV

7. Which of the following statements about neurons with a myelin sheath is TRUE? 7.____

   A. They transmit nerve impulses rapidly.
   B. They consist of multiple cell bodies.
   C. Once an axon is damaged, it can't be repaired.
   D. Neurotransmitters may be involved in transmitting a message, but are not required.

8. Which of the following is consistent with a stroke involving the left posterior cerebellar artery? 8.____

   A. diplopia
   B. uniform visual hallucinations
   C. memory impairment
   D. aphasia

9. Which of the following is LEAST likely to be involved in a cran-iopharyngioma? 9.____

   A. hypothalamus
   B. optic nerve
   C. third ventricle
   D. pituitary gland

10. The pons and reticular formation are found in the 10.____

    A. spinal cord
    B. forebrain
    C. midbrain
    D. hindbrain

11. Tricyclic antidepressants effect neurotransmitters during 11.____

    A. degradation
    B. storage
    C. reuptake
    D. production

12. Impulses are transmitted by motor neurons 12.____

    A. among components of the central nervous system
    B. from stimulus receptors
    C. away from the central nervous system
    D. between the axon bulbs of individual neurons

13. Cubital tunnel syndrome is characterized by each of the following, EXCEPT 13.____

A. weakness in intrinsic hand muscles
B. parasthesia/numbness in ring finger
C. negative elbow flexion test
D. medial elbow pain

14. Which of the following neoplasms is well-differentiated, likely to present with hydrocephalus, and more common in children? 14.____

A. Brain stem glioma
B. Ependymoma
C. Choroid plexus papilloma
D. Meningioma

15. During the ______, an action potential cannot be gener-ated in a neuron. 15.____

A. membrane hyperpolarization
B. membrane depolarization
C. relative refractory period
D. absolute refractory period

16. An electrical synapse is also known as a(n) 16.____

A. ligand-gated channel
B. voltage-gated channel
C. gap junction channel
D. transmitter-gated channel

17. In cases of cerebral edema, the greatest increases in sodium and water content typically occur in the 17.____

A. white matter
B. meninges
C. gray matter
D. dura

18. What is the term for the innermost layer of the meninges? 18.____

A. arachnoid
B. falx
C. pia mater
D. dura mater

19. A 50-year-old man has experienced severe headaches that have wors-ened over the past several weeks, and now has difficulty moving his left arm. He presents papilledema that is worse on the right. The most likely condition to be associated with these findings is 19.____

A. neovascularization around a glioma
B. HIV encephalopathy
C. neuronal storage disease
D. overproduction of cerebrospinal fluid

20. The cerebral lobes primarily involved in planning and performing movement are the _______ lobes. 20.___

A. temporal
B. parietal
C. sagittal
D. frontal

21. A person has lost pain and temperature sensation, but has retained the sensation of touch. A disorder consistent with these findings is 21.___

A. Cerebrovascular accident
B. Syringomyelia
C. Subdural hemotoma
D. Wegener's granulomatosis

22. Which of the following disorders is associated with a reduction in the size of the caudate nuclei? 22.___

A. Parkinson's disease
B. Huntington's disease
C. Charcot-Marie-Tooth disease
D. Amyotrophic lateral sclerosis

23. In the vestibular system, rotations of the head are sensed by the 23.___

A. ipsilateral and contralateral neurons of the brain stem
B. maculae of the utricle and the saccule
C. ampullae in the semicircular canals
D. Y nucleus

24. Typical findings of carpal tunnel syndrome include each of the following, EXCEPT 24.___

A. decreased sensation in the thumb
B. atrophy of thenar eminence
C. spasms of the flexor carpi ulnaris
D. decreased sensation in the index and middle fingers

25. The earliest symptom of acoustic nerve tumors is usually 25.___

A. hemiparesis
B. vertigo
C. ataxia
D. tinnitus

KEY (CORRECT ANSWERS)

1. C
2. A
3. B
4. B
5. B
6. A
7. A
8. B
9. A
10. D
11. C
12. C
13. C
14. C
15. D
16. C
17. A
18. C
19. A
20. D
21. B
22. B
23. C
24. C
25. D

TEST 2

DIRECTIONS: Each question or incomplete statement is followed by several suggested answers or completions. Select the one the BEST answers the question or completes the statement. *PRINT THE LETTER OF THE CORRECT ANSWER IN THE SPACE AT THE RIGHT.*

1. Which of the following is a disorder caused by excessive cerebrospinal fluid? 1.____

   A. Meningitis
   B. Hydrocephalus
   C. Subdural edema
   D. Pneumoencephalus

2. The main classes of neuroreceptors include each of the following, EXCEPT 2.____

   A. photoreceptors
   B. nociceptors
   C. mechanoreceptors
   D. palpireceptors

3. Which of the following is NOT associated with central vertigo? 3.____

   A. Multiple sclerosis
   B. Vascular insufficiency
   C. Meniere's disease
   D. Migraine headache

4. A patient has subacute lower back pain, suspected nerve involvement represented by leg pain should be evaluated by means of 4.____

   A. CAT scan
   B. electromyelography
   C. knee-jerk reflex test
   D. MRI scan

5. Which of the following are receptor-blocking drugs used to treat the psychotic symptoms of schizophrenia? 5.____

   A. Phenothiazines
   B. Menzodiazepines
   C. Oxidase inhibitors
   D. Atropines

6. The main function of the sodium/potassium pump is to 6.____

   A. polarize the neuron
   B. release neurotransmitter
   C. maintain cell volume
   D. decode the strength of a stimulus

7. Which of the following neoplasms is likely to be located in the 4th ventricle in childhood, or in the spinal cord in adults? 7.____

A. Oligodendroglioma
B. Ependymoma
C. Glioblastoma
D. Astrocytoma

8. Major causes of dementia include 8.____

I. cephalic disorders
II. Alzheimer's disease
III. multi-infarct
IV. metabolic disorders

A. I and II
B. II and III
C. II and IV
D. I, II, III and IV

9. Tay-Sachs disease is associated with a decrease in 9.____

A. gamma globulin
B. sphingomyelinase
C. hexosaminidase A
D. glucocerebrosidase

10. Which of the following areas would NOT be involved in a basilar artery stroke? 10.____

A. Pons
B. Midbrain
C. Basal ganglia
D. Occipital cortex

11. A seizure lasting more than 10 minutes, or a second seizure prior to regaining consciousness from a first seizure, is defined as 11.____

A. generalized
B. tonic-clonic
C. complex partial
D. status epilepticus

12. Common symptoms of frontal lobe tumors include 12.____

I. hemiplegia
II. seizures
III. memory deficit
IV. speech disturbances

A. I only
B. I, II and III
C. II, III and IV
D. I, II, III and IV

13. Berry aneurysms occur at the 13.____

A. lacunae
B. posterior pericallosal artery
C. basilar artery
D. bifurcation of the Circle of Willis

14. Of the following conditions, which is LEAST likely to obstruct the flow of cerebrospinal fluid and cause ventricular enlargement? 14.____

A. pneumococcal meningitis
B. epidural hematoma
C. forking in the aqueduct of Sylvius
D. intraventricular hemorrhage

15. The lateral geniculate is a thalamic nucleus involved in 15.____

A. vision
B. hearing
C. taste
D. smell

16. Gangliogliomas are rare neoplasms that usually affect the ______ lobes of the cerebral hemispheres. 16.____

A. frontal
B. temporal
C. parietal
D. occipital

17. A hemorrhage involving the region of the right basal ganglia is most likely to develop as a result of 17.____

A. severe trauma
B. vascular malformation
C. hypertension
D. encephalitis

18. Most motor neurons are stimulated by 18.____

A. mechanoreceptors
B. sensory neurons
C. glands
D. interneurons

19. A 53-year-old woman has diabetes mellitus. Which of the following is LEAST likely to be associated with her peripheral neuropathy? 19.____

A. Symmetrical involvement
B. More severe effect on axons than dendrites
C. More severe effect on motor nerves than sensory nerves
D. More severe effect on distal nerves in the extremities

20. Electrochemical equilibrium refers to the balance between ______ force and ______ force. 20.____

A. nuclear; inertial
B. electrostatic; diffusion
C. molecular; electromagnetic
D. frictional; gravitational

21. The brain's third ventricle is surrounded by the 21.____

A. hypothalamus
B. thalamus
C. aqueduct of Sylvius
D. pons

22. A neurons action potential 22.____

I. appears on the cell body membrane
II. is "all-or-none"
III. is self-generating
IV. uses volt-sensitive ion channels

A. I and IV
B. I, II and III
C. II, III and IV
D. I, II, III and IV

23. Rods and cones are examples of 23.____

I. chemoreceptors
II. proprioceptors
III. photoreceptors
IV. exteroceptors

A. I only
B. I and II
C. III only
D. III and IV

24. The cerebellum negotiates 24.____

A. emotions
B. somatosensory input
C. speech
D. motor coordination

25. Causes of sensorineural hearing loss include 25.____

I. congenital
II. Meniere's disease
III. aging
IV. acoustic injury

A. I only
B. I, III and IV
C. II and III
D. I, II, III and IV

KEY (CORRECT ANSWERS)

1. B
2. D
3. C
4. B
5. A

6. C
7. B
8. B
9. C
10. C

11. D
12. B
13. D
14. A
15. A

16. B
17. C
18. D
19. C
20. B

21. B
22. C
23. C
24. D
25. D

TEST 3

DIRECTIONS: Each question or incomplete statement is followed by several suggested answers or completions. Select the one the BEST answers the question or completes the statement. *PRINT THE LETTER OF THE CORRECT ANSWER IN THE SPACE AT THE RIGHT.*

1. The frequency of "treatable" causes of dementia is estimated to be about ______%. 1.____

   A. 20
   B. 40
   C. 60
   D. 80

2. Which of the following is NOT a type of glioma? 2.____

   A. Ependymoma
   B. Astrocytoma
   C. Oligodendroglioma
   D. Chordoma

3. The central nervous system interprets impulses based on their frequency and 3.____

   A. origin
   B. speed
   C. type
   D. duration

4. The ion responsible for the reversal of membrane potential during the action potential is 4.____

   A. calcium
   B. chloride
   C. sodium
   D. potassium

5. Which of the following is NOT a common symptom of Horner's syndrome? 5.____

   A. Red, dry skin (anhidrosis)
   B. Drooping eyelid (ptosis)
   C. Tinnitus
   D. Pupil constriction (miosis)

6. Each of the following senses is processed in the thalamus before reaching the cerebral cortex, EXCEPT 6.____

   A. taste
   B. smell
   C. vision
   D. somatosensory

7. Eye movement is governed by which of the following cranial nerves? 7.____

   A. second (optic)
   B. fifth (trigeminal)
   C. sixth (abducent)
   D. eighth (vestibulocochlear)

8. An embolism that causes acute onset of left hemiparesis, facial droop, and occlusion of the right middle cerebral artery has come from the 8.____

A. aortic arch
B. saphenous vein
C. carotid bifurcation
D. left atrium

9. The strength of a stimulus is typically encoded in the 9.____

A. frequency of the action potentials that it generates
B. voltage of the postsynaptic membrane
C. number of action potentials that it generates
D. threshold voltage of the neuron

10. Which of the following neoplasms is ALWAYS located in the cerebellum? 10.____

A. Oligodendroglioma
B. Meningioma
C. Schwannoma
D. Medulloblastoma

11. A seizure that arises in both cerebral hemispheres is described as 11.____

A. complex
B. febrile
C. tonic-clonic
D. generalized

12. Metachromatic leukodystrophy is associated with a deficiency in 12.____

A. myrosinase
B. glucocerebrosidase
C. neuraminidase
D. sphingomyelinase

13. Inhibitory neurotransmitters 13.____

A. raise the threshold voltage of the neuron
B. open sodium channels in the plasma membrane
C. hyperpolarize the postsynaptic membrane
D. depolarize the postsynaptic membrane

14. Dymyelinating diseases include 14.____

I. metachromatic leukodystrophy
II. postinfectious encephalomyelitis
III. multiple sclerosis
IV. progressive multifocal leukoencephalopathy

A. I and II
B. I, III and IV
C. II and III
D. I, II, III and IV

15. A 50-year-old woman has had a severe headache for several days. A physical exam reveals right-side papilledema, and a head CAT scan reveals a marked right-to-left midline shift. An MRI scan shows a 5 cm enhancing mass lesion in the right parietal region with marked surrounding edema. Which of the following conditions is most likely? 15.____

A. Pontine hemorrhages
B. Diffuse subarachnoid hemorrhage
C. Posterior cerebral artery thrombosis
D. Superior sagittal sinus thrombosis

16. The hemispheres of the cerebrum are separated by the 16.____

A. superior sagittal sinus
B. falx cerebri
C. choroid plexus
D. tentorium cerebri

17. Alzheimer's disease is characterized by each of the following, EXCEPT 17.____

A. Neuritic plaques
B. Hirano bodies
C. decreased myelin
D. decreased numbers of neurons in the nucleus basalis of Meynert

18. What area of the brain is implicated in long-term potentiation? 18.____

A. Hypothalamus
B. Hippocampus
C. Amygdala
D. Pons

19. Axons are specialized structures that are designed to 19.____

A. conduct electrical impulses
B. interpret electrical messages
C. generate chemical messages
D. protect nerve cells

20. Symptoms of a basilar artery stroke include 20.____

I. visual field deficits
II. quadriparesis
III. diplopia
IV. right homonymous hemianopsia

A. I only
B. I, II and III
C. II and III
D. I, II, III and IV

21. Motor neuron axons travel outward from the spinal cord through the 21.____

A. cauda equina
B. dorsal root
C. ventral root
D. medial root

22. Parietal lobe tumors are most likely to be associated with 22.____

A. a loss of the ability to write (agraphia)
B. aphasia
C. ataxia
D. hemiparesis

23. Which of the following would be sensed by an exteroceptor? 23.____

A. Muscle tension
B. Smell
C. Lung inflation
D. Mechanical pain

24. A stroke involving the right middle cerebral artery is LEAST likely to affect the 24.____

A. basal ganglia
B. internal brain capsule
C. parietal cortex
D. pons

25. Which of the following is LEAST likely to occur as a consequence of severe head trauma? 25.____

A. Cerebral edema
B. Loss of sense of smell
C. Subdural hematoma
D. Cerebral vasculitis

KEY (CORRECT ANSWERS)

1. A
2. D
3. A
4. C
5. C
6. B
7. C
8. D
9. A
10. D
11. D
12. B
13. C
14. D
15. A
16. B
17. C
18. B
19. A
20. B
21. C
22. A
23. D
24. D
25. D

EXAMINATION SECTION
TEST 1

DIRECTIONS: Each question or incomplete statement is followed by several suggested answers or completions. Select the one the BEST answers the question or completes the statement. *PRINT THE LETTER OF THE CORRECT ANSWER IN THE SPACE AT THE RIGHT.*

1. A neuron's action potential is usually generated in the 1.____

   A. cell body
   B. axon hillock
   C. nucleus
   D. Schwann cell

2. Classical manifestations of neuroleptic malignant syndrome include each of the following, EXCEPT 2.____

   A. Resting tremor
   B. Hyperthermia
   C. Hypertonic skeletal muscles
   D. Fluctuating consciousness

3. The basal ganglia regulates ______ functions. 3.____

   A. auditory
   B. somatosensory
   C. motor
   D. visual

4. Cluster headaches are characterized by each of the following, EXCEPT 4.____

   A. Periorbital pain
   B. Nasal congestion
   C. Photosensitivity
   D. Homolateral redness of eye, nose

5. Somatic neural sensations originate from receptors in 5.____

   A. a specific location in the body
   B. muscles
   C. more than one location in the body
   D. tactile zones in the hands and feet

6. A 46-year-old man develops a psychosis and a choreiform movement disorder. The most likely condition is 6.____

   A. Creutzfeld-Jakov disease
   B. Alzheimer's disease
   C. Huntington's disease
   D. Multiple sclerosis

7. A child is stillborn at 34 weeks with marked hydrops fetalis, organomegaly, extensive cerebral necrosis, and preventricular calcification. The cause of death was most likely 7.____

A. cytomegalovirus
B. HIV
C. Epstein-Barr virus
D. Herpes simplex virus

8. The ion necessary for the release of a neurotransmitter is 8.____

A. potassium
B. sodium
C. chloride
D. calcium

9. Emotions and problem-solving are associated with the brain's _______ lobes. 9.____

A. frontal
B. parietal
C. temporal
D. occipital

10. The graded potentials of a sensory receptor are collectively as 10.____

A. Excitatory postsynaptic potential (EPSP)
B. Inhibitory postsynaptic potential (IPSP)
C. Generator potential
D. Threshold

11. "Cushing's Triad" refers to three findings consistent with intracranial pressure. Which of the following is NOT one of these findings? 11.____

A. Irregular breathing
B. Delirium
C. Hypertension
D. Bradycardia

12. A 48-year-old man has become comatose. He has right-side papille-dema and cerebellar tonsillar herniation. Which of the following conditions is LEAST likely? 12.____

A. Glioblastoma multiforme
B. Chronic subdural hematoma
C. Wernicke's disease
D. Cerebral abscess

13. The classic set of symptoms of Meniere's disease includes each of the following, EXCEPT 13.____

A. Tinnitus
B. Hearing loss
C. Vertigo
D. Numbness or tingling in the extremities

14. The ventral amygdalofugal pathway carries projections from the amygdala to the cingulate cortex and the 14.____

    A. lateral hypothalamus
    B. orbitofrontal cortex
    C. diencephalon
    D. temporal cortex

15. Of the following brain neoplasms, which has the best post-surgical prognosis? 15.____

    A. Schwannoma
    B. Medulloblastoma
    C. Glioblastoma multiforme
    D. Astrocytoma

16. A neurotransmitter allows negatively charged chloride ions into the neuron and increases the membrane potential. Which of the following has occurred? 16.____

    A. Facilitated diffusion
    B. Inhibitory postsynaptic potential (IPSP)
    C. Excitatory postsynaptic potential (EPSP)
    D. Threshold voltage

17. Which of the following types of brain neoplasms is LEAST common among children? 17.____

    A. Medulloblastoma
    B. Ependymoma
    C. Astrocytoma
    D. Meningioma

18. What is the term for a single neuron's transmission of an impulse to many neurons? 18.____

    A. Radiation
    B. Refraction
    C. Summation
    D. Divergence

19. Approximately what percentage of cerebrovascular accidents are hemorrhagic? 19.____

    A. 20-30
    B. 30-50
    C. 50-70
    D. 70-80

20. Most commonly, subarachnoid hemorrhages occur secondary to 20.____

    A. blood dyscrasias and respiratory problems
    B. cerebral neoplasms
    C. acute infection
    D. arteriovenous malformations (AVM) or berry aneurysm rupture

21. Which of the following would be sensed by an interoceptor? 21.___

A. Joint angle
B. Venous pressure
C. Thermal pain
D. Linear acceleration

22. Which of the following is LEAST likely to be associated with Duret hemorrhages of the midbrain and/or the pons subsequent to severe uncal herniation? 22.___

A. Hypertensive hemorrhage
B. Alzheimer's disease
C. Severe head trauma
D. Meningioma

23. The most prominent example of cortical commissural fibers is the 23.___

A. posterior commissure
B. choroid plexus
C. corpus callosum
D. falx cerebri

24. Which of the following disorders is characterized by a loss of myelin in the central nervous system? 24.___

A. Amyotrophic lateral sclerosis (ALS)
B. Myasthenia gravis (MG)
C. Charcot-Marie-Tooth (CMT) disease
D. Multiple sclerosis (MS)

25. Occipital lobe tumors are most likely to be associated with 25.___

A. blindness in one direction (hemianopsia)
B. loss of a sense of smell (anosmia)
C. mental or personality changes
D. memory deficit

KEY (CORRECT ANSWERS)

1. B
2. A
3. C
4. C
5. C
6. C
7. A
8. D
9. A
10. C
11. B
12. C
13. D
14. B
15. A
16. B
17. D
18. D
19. A
20. D
21. B
22. B
23. C
24. D
25. A

TEST 2

DIRECTIONS: Each question or incomplete statement is followed by several suggested answers or completions. Select the one the BEST answers the question or completes the statement. *PRINT THE LETTER OF THE CORRECT ANSWER IN THE SPACE AT THE RIGHT.*

1. The majority of the brain is made up of 1.____

   A. sensory neurons
   B. motor neurons
   C. somatosensory receptors
   D. interneurons

2. Each of the following types of seizures involves an alteration of consciousness, EXCEPT 2.____

   A. complex partial
   B. absence
   C. simple partial
   D. temporal lobe

3. If a patient's history and physical examination reveal a significant chance that headache symptoms are secondary to a brain stem lesion, the most appropriate diagnostic tool is 3.____

   A. MRI scan
   B. electromyelography
   C. CAT scan
   D. Rorschach test

4. What is the term for the mechanoreceptors of the ear? 4.____

   A. Hair cells
   B. Cochlear cells
   C. Proprioceptors
   D. Vestibular cells

5. The origins of the 5th, 6th, 7th, and 8th cranial nerves are contained within the 5.____

   A. pons
   B. cerebellum
   C. medulla oblongata
   D. limbic system

6. "Silent" brain tumors – those presenting no symptoms – are most likely to arise in the _______ lobe. 6.____

   A. frontal
   B. parietal
   C. temporal
   D. occipital

7. Which of the following is NOT a part of the limbic system? 7.____

   A. Substantia nigra
   B. Cingulate gyrus
   C. Amygdala
   D. Septum

8. Bell's palsy is a neurological disorder caused by damage to the 8.____

   A. fourth cranial (trochlear) nerve
   B. sixth cranial (abducent) nerve
   C. seventh cranial (facial) nerve
   D. eighth cranial (vestibulocochlear) nerve

9. A 30-year old man suffers an acute onset of confusion, followed by a seizure. A CAT scan reveals lesion in the left temporal lobe. The findings are most likely to be associated with 9.____

   A. astrocytoma
   B. papovavirus
   C. herpes simplex virus
   D. berry aneurysm

10. A proprioceptor is capable of sensing 10.____

    A. taste
    B. arterial blood pressure
    C. muscle tension
    D. hair movement

11. A 41-year old woman reports difficulty chewing and swallowing, along with fatigue that worsens with exercise and improves with rest. She presents with drooping eyelids. These findings are consistent with 11.____

    A. Guillain-Barre syndrome
    B. myasthenia gravis
    C. neurofibromatosis
    D. fibromyalgia

12. Each of the following is associated with degenerative neurologic diseases, EXCEPT 12.____

    A. lack of targeted or curative treatments
    B. worsening neurologic deficits over many years
    C. acute symptoms from a mass effect
    D. loss of specific neuronal groups

13. During impulse transmission, the voltage-gated sodium channels of myelinated neurons are confined to 13.____

    A. Schwann cells
    B. the axon hillock
    C. nodes of Ranvier
    D. excitatory synapses

14. The release of acetylcholine can be inhibited by introducing the toxin 14.____

    A. botulin B. tetanus C. globulin D. selenium

15. Which of the following is MOST likely to be found with a fast-growing left hemispheric glioma? 15.___

A. Subdural hematoma
B. Basal ganglia hemorrhage
C. Pontine Duret hemorrhage
D. Subarachnoid hemorrhage

16. Sulci 16.___

A. separate the cerebrum from the cerebellum
B. are furrows in the cerebral cortex
C. line the cerebral ventricles
D. are fluids in the inner ear

17. Approximately what percentage of patients with multiple sclerosis will develop optic neuritis? 17.___

A. 20   B. 40   C. 60   D. 80

18. Which of the following types of brain neoplasms is LEAST common among adults? 18.___

A. Ependymoma
B. Glioblastoma multiforme
C. Metastatic tumors
D. Meningioma

19. Within a neuron, graded potentials 19.___

A. produce graded action potentials
B. may aggregate in space and time
C. usually hyperpolarize the membrane
D. always produce action potentials

20. Diseases of the motor neurons include 20.___

I. Amyotrophic lateral sclerosis
II. Charcot-Marie-Tooth (CMT) disease
III. Werndig-Hoffman diseases
IV. Huntington's Disease

A. I only   B. I and III   C. II, III and IV   D. IV only

21. A subdural hematoma typically occurs 21.___

A. between the dura and the skull
B. secondary to a rupture of the bridging veins of the brain
C. secondary to a fracture of the temporal bone
D. between the cranium and the scalp

22. At the emergency room, a 7-year-old child is listless, has a temperature of 100.6° F, and presents nuchal rigidity. A lumbar puncture yields slightly cloudy cerebrospinal fluid with elevated protein and decreased glucose. A culture of this fluid will most likely yield 22.____

A. aspergillus fumigatus
B. cryptococcus neoformans
C. streptococcus pneumoniae
D. hemophilus influenzae

23. The brain is divided into upper and lower parts by the ______ section. 23.____

A. horizontal
B. sagittal
C. coronal
D. ipsilateral

24. Which of the following is a drug used exclusively in the treatment of absence seizures? 24.____

A. Diazepam
B. Ethosuxamide
C. Phenobarbital
D. Phenytoin (Dilantin)

25. A 48-year-old man has experienced right-sided headaches for nearly 6 years, and has recently noted some weakness in his left hand. A CAT scan shows a well-defined lateral mass that is compressing the right hemisphere in the frontal-parietal area. Most likely, this mass is a(n) 25.____

A. meningioma
B. glioblastoma multiform
C. Schwannoma
D. astrocytoma

KEY (CORRECT ANSWERS)

1. D
2. C
3. A
4. A
5. A
6. C
7. A
8. C
9. C
10. C
11. B
12. C
13. C
14. A
15. C
16. B
17. B
18. A
19. B
20. B
21. B
22. D
23. A
24. B
25. A

TEST 3

DIRECTIONS: Each question or incomplete statement is followed by several suggested answers or completions. Select the one the BEST answers the question or completes the statement. *PRINT THE LETTER OF THE CORRECT ANSWER IN THE SPACE AT THE RIGHT.*

1. A person experiencing nausea, vomiting, tinnitus, or hearing loss, accompanied by horizontal or rotary nystagmus, is experiencing ______ vertigo. 1.____

   A. migraine
   B. central
   C. peripheral
   D. vascular insufficiency

2. The forebrain is also known as the 2.____

   A. tela choroidea
   B. prosencephalon
   C. superior colliculus
   D. diencephalon

3. Which of the following disorders is associated with pink Lewy bodies? 3.____

   A. Huntington's disease
   B. Alzheimer's disease
   C. Creutzfeld-Jakov disease
   D. Parkinson's disease

4. Which of the following is the location where sound waves are converted to nerve impulses? 4.____

   A. Vestibular system
   B. Inner ear
   C. Middle ear
   D. Brain stem

5. An 82-year-old woman suffers ischemic injury with cerebral infarction. A few days later, it is most likely that the cerebrum will yield a histo-pathological finding of ______ necrosis. 5.____

   A. liquefactive
   B. fat necrosis
   C. coagulative
   D. gangrenous

6. Which of the following is NOT found in the midbrain? 6.____

   A. Cerebral peduncle
   B. Inferior colliculus
   C. Tegmentum
   D. Tectum

7. The "triad of Wernicke-Korsakoff syndrome" includes each of the following, EXCEPT 7.____

A. ophthalmoplegia
B. aphasia
C. ataxia
D. psychosis

8. Wallerian degeneration of a peripheral nerve can 8.____

I. be seen in Guillain-Barre syndrome
II. can occur when the neuron that controls an axon dies
III. can be followed by regeneration
IV. can occur following severe trauma or infarction

A. I and II
B. II, III and IV
C. III and IV
D. I, II, III and IV

9. The theory that all the neurons in the body are physically connected is the _______ hypothesis. 9.____

A. coalition
B. reticular
C. connectivity
D. associative

10. Approximately two-thirds of people with epilepsy have _______ seizures. 10.____

A. tonic-clonic
B. generalized absence
C. status epilepticus
D. complex partial

11. The brain's _______ lobe is involved in the understanding of visual images and the meaning of written words. 11.____

A. frontal
B. parietal
C. temporal
D. occipital

12. Which of the following is NOT consistent with a stroke involving the right middle cerebral artery? 12.____

A. Spatial disorientation
B. Left hemiparesis
C. Aphasia
D. Hemianopsia

13. Wernicke-Korsakoff syndrome affects the 13.____

I. thalamus
II. mamillary bodies
III. amygdala

A. I only
B. I and II
C. II only
D. I, II and III

14. Epinephrine is a 14.____

A. neuropeptide
B. neurotransmitter
C. neuron
D. neurotoxin

15. The postcentral gyrus is a cerebral structure that serves as a(n) ______ cortex. 15.____

A. visual
B. olfactory
C. somatosensory
D. motor

16. Which of the following is MOST likely to be associated with hypertensive arteriosclerosis? 16.____

A. Epidural hematoma
B. Subarachnoid hemorrhage
C. Subdural hematoma
D. Basal ganglia hemorrhage

17. During a radical mastectomy involving a 69-year-old patient, the anesthesiologist reports a drop in blood pressure. If hypotension lasts longer than 30 minutes, the most likely consequence is 17.____

A. parietal lobe hemorrhagic infarct
B. anterior pituitary necrosis
C. lacunar infarcts of basal ganglia
D. linear parasagittal infarction

18. What is the function of neuroglial cells? 18.____

A. Supporting and protecting neurons
B. Receiving chemical messages
C. Regulating sodium/potassium levels
D. Regenerating damaged nerve cell bodies

19. Symptoms of central vertigo can be described as 19.____

I. more subtle and less intense than peripheral vertigo
II. insidious in onset
III. usually difficult for the patient to explain
IV. occasionally including vertical nystagmus

A. I only
B. I and II
C. III only
D. I, II, III and IV

20. Common symptoms of brain stem neoplasms include each of the following, EXCEPT 20.____

A. dysphagia
B. vomiting
C. tinnitus
D. ataxia

21. The point at which graded potentials in a neuron reach an action potential is known as the 21.____

A. excitatory postsynaptic potential (EPSP)
B. inhibitory postsynaptic potential (IPSP)
C. threshold voltage
D. refractory period

22. Which of the following is LEAST likely to be associated with neural syphilis? 22.____

A. Hemorrhagic encephalitis
B. Spinal cord dorsal column atrophy
C. Endarteritis
D. Chronic meningitis

23. The risk of stroke for a patient with a history of transient ischemic attacks is about ______ % per year and ______ % after five years. 23.____

A. 5; 25
B. 10; 33
C. 20; 20
D. 33; 66

24. The most common site of a central nervous system lymphoma is 24.____

A. the cerebellum
B. the pons
C. the spinal cord
D. one of the cerebral hemispheres

25. The sympathetic and parasympathetic nervous systems are immediate divisions of the ______ nervous system. 25.____

A. vestibular
B. autonomic
C. central
D. peripheral

KEY (CORRECT ANSWERS)

1. C
2. B
3. D
4. B
5. A

6. D
7. B
8. B
9. B
10. D

11. D
12. C
13. B
14. B
15. C

16. D
17. D
18. A
19. D
20. C

21. C
22. A
23. B
24. D
25. B

EXAMINATION SECTION
TEST 1

DIRECTIONS: Each question or incomplete statement is followed by several suggested answers or completions. Select the one that BEST answers the question or completes the statement. *PRINT THE LETTER OF THE CORRECT ANSWER IN THE SPACE AT THE RIGHT.*

1. Discerning the common elements in situations that are otherwise different is referred to as 1.____

   A. cue reduction
   B. discrimination
   C. relevant grouping
   D. generalizing
   E. abstracting

2. Closed system thinking is BEST illustrated by 2.____

   A. solving a series of addition problems
   B. determining the best route to a new location
   C. writing a novel
   D. devising a new formula
   E. inventing a better mousetrap

3. Distribution of practice is especially relevant to 3.____

   A. weakening of incorrect responses
   B. slowing down performance
   C. increased tension
   D. reducing accuracy of performance
   E. reducing motivation

4. Directive therapy may be BEST described as a therapy in which 4.____

   A. the subject selects his own goals
   B. past experiences are given primary attention in problem solving
   C. the therapist prescribes
   D. the individual, not the present problem, is the focus
   E. the emotional rather than intellectual factors are emphasized

5. Drugs which produce behavior resembling psychoses are called 5.____

   A. psychotherapeutic drugs
   B. tranquilizers
   C. sulfa-drugs
   D. antibiotics
   E. psychotomimetic drugs

6. A characteristic wave pattern of waking-sleeping is shown by the record made by a 6.____

   A. compass
   B. thermometer
   C. kymograph
   D. galvanometer
   E. electroencephalograph

7. A woman with strong maternal tendencies is found incapable of bearing children and is in no position to adopt one. The behavior that would be MOST valuable to her is 7.____

   A. sublimation
   B. rationalization
   C. regression
   D. projection
   E. fantasy

8. That part of the process of concept formation where the individual learns to respond only to certain properties that objects have in common is called 8.____

A. differentiation B. assimilation C. abstraction
D. generalization E. adaptation

9. An abscissa would be found in 9.____

A. the nervous system
B. the eye
C. a human ear
D. the reactions of a schizophrenic
E. a graph

10. Genes for blue eyes are said to be recessive. Mr. and Mrs. Jones have blue eyes. If they have eight children, the number having blue eyes should be 10.____

A. 6 B. 2 C. 4 D. 8 E. 0

11. The subjectively established unit of measure of visual intensity is called 11.____

A. bril B. fissure C. pyknic D. veg E. rho

12. Stating that a mental disorder is functional means that it 12.____

A. can best be treated by surgery or drugs
B. is concerned with the personality only
C. is a product of imagination only
D. has been learned
E. produces no physical symptoms

13. A temporary flat place in a learning curve is called 13.____

A. a fatigue index B. an ordinate
C. a plateau D. an abscissa
E. skewedness

14. An experimental procedure which involves reinforcement of one stimulus and extinction of all others will eventually lead to 14.____

A. generalization
B. latent learning
C. higher order conditioning
D. conditioned discrimination
E. negative adaptation

15. The refractory period has reference to 15.____

A. nerve functioning B. retroactive inhibition
C. reverberating circuits D. regressive tendencies
E. retinal images

16. Self-understanding is aided MOST by 16.____

A. repressing threatening memories
B. attempting to understand one's own motives
C. the use of defense mechanisms

D. avoiding anxiety-producing situations
E. venting one's emotions whenever one feels like it

17. Ossicles are found in the 17.____

A. kidneys B. eyes C. heart D. ears E. lungs

18. The MOST important factor in producing apparent motion in the absence of actual motion is 18.____

A. time interval between stimuli
B. fatigue
C. size of stimuli
D. intensity of stimuli
E. actual movement of stimuli

19. Negative transfer of training means that when something has been previously learned, it 19.____

A. hinders recall
B. reinforces new learning
C. makes one forget old learning
D. aids learning in a new situation
E. hinders new learning

20. Mrs. Jones did not want her third child and has never been able to really care about it, but she shows excessive affection toward the child. 20.____
This is an example of

A. rationalization
B. repression
C. sublimation
D. reaction formation
E. projection

21. The SIMPLEST form of learning is generally regarded as a form of 21.____

A. conditioning
B. rote memory
C. associative process
D. functional learning
E. discrimination

22. A defense mechanism MOST apt to do harm to others is that of 22.____

A. rationalization
B. reaction formation
C. compensation
D. projection
E. sublimation

23. The term insanity as viewed by the psychological world 23.____

A. is synonymous with neurosis
B. is synonymous with psychosis
C. is a legal term
D. means disorganization of the ego structure
E. refers to loss of contact with reality

24. When the brain is exposed and the somesthetic area is stimulated directly by a micro-electrode, subjects report no pain since pain is 24.____

A. an abnormal condition
B. a function of the thalamus

C. not a brain function
D. a product of the imagination
E. a function of the cortex

25. There would be no galvanic skin reflex if there were 25.____

A. no sweat gland activity
B. no cortical stimulation
C. damage to the occipital lobe
D. no creative thought
E. no reminiscence

KEY (CORRECT ANSWERS)

1. E
2. A
3. A
4. C
5. E

6. E
7. A
8. C
9. E
10. D

11. A
12. D
13. C
14. D
15. A

16. B
17. D
18. A
19. E
20. D

21. A
22. D
23. C
24. B
25. A

TEST 2

DIRECTIONS: Each question or incomplete statement is followed by several suggested answers or completions. Select the one that BEST answers the question or completes the statement. *PRINT THE LETTER OF THE CORRECT ANSWER IN THE SPACE AT THE RIGHT.*

1. Persons who hold prejudices against minority groups MOST likely retain their negative attitudes as a result of 1.____

   A. proven inferiority of minority groups
   B. wide reading and studying
   C. general distrust or dislike of persons who are different
   D. personal experiences
   E. logical thinking

2. The temporary nature of the extinction of a previously conditioned response is BEST exemplified by 2.____

   A. relearning
   B. stimulus generalization
   C. conditioned discrimination
   D. spontaneous recovery
   E. higher order conditioning

3. Putting two or more elements of past experience together to make something new is called 3.____

   A. differentiation
   B. reasoning
   C. abstracting
   D. learning set
   E. solution by reduced cues

4. The simultaneous contraction and relaxation of antagonistic muscles is called 4.____

   A. reciprocal inhibition
   B. general inhibition
   C. extension reflex
   D. reflex action
   E. flexion reflex

5. Pavlov's experiments in which he used one conditioned response to build another conditioned response is an example of 5.____

   A. secondary conditioning
   B. higher-order conditioning
   C. classical conditioning
   D. reinforcement
   E. advanced conditioning

6. If a child born does not have enough oxygen for a long period of time, or has no oxygen at all for a short period of time, and still lives, he is likely to 6.____

   A. become extremely active in early childhood
   B. become an invalid
   C. recover completely in a long time

D. recover completely in a short time
E. have a marked loss in intelligence

7. In emotional states, the sympathetic part of the autonomic nervous system 7.____

A. reduces the discharge of adrenalin
B. decreases heart rate
C. causes irregular breathing
D. contracts the pupil of the eye
E. speeds up the flow of saliva

8. A defense mechanism is a device adopted unconsciously by the individual 8.____

A. in order to achieve beyond his level of aspiration
B. for the deception of authority figures
C. so that he may solve his basic problems
D. so that he may engage in fantasy
E. for fooling himself about his motivational conflicts

9. We can expect to find the MOST elaborate social structures in 9.____

A. societies with few natural resources
B. highly industrialized societies
C. societies with strict child-rearing techniques
D. primitive societies
E. the oldest cultures

10. A regression to childish levels of behavior occurs in a type of schizophrenia called 10.____

A. hebephrenic
B. dementia praecox
C. simple
D. paranoid
E. catatonic

11. Letters of recommendation when used for selecting employees are usually regarded as being 11.____

A. unbiased evaluations of employees
B. of doubtful value
C. highly reliable
D. rarely stereotyped
E. good discriminators between qualified and unqualified persons

12. One of the MOST obvious characteristics of perception is its 12.____

A. resistance to shifting
B. all inclusive quality
C. agreement with the physical world
D. selective nature
E. unique sameness from person to person

13. In the conditioning experiments of Pavlov with the dog, bell, and food, the dependent variable was the 13.____

A. condition of the dog
B. amount of salivation
C. time element
D. ringing of the bell
E. presenting of food

14. We could not form concepts if we could not 14.____

A. see colors
B. vocalize
C. read
D. discriminate
E. form clear mental images

15. The use of psychological methods and techniques by employers to select and retain the BEST employees is a branch of psychology known as ______ psychology. 15.____

A. social
B. industrial
C. general
D. vocational
E. clinical

16. One of Freud's MAIN contributions to psychology was 16.____

A. the classification of mental disorders
B. his theory of personality
C. the use of the experimental method
D. the use of scientific techniques
E. his use of phenomenology

17. The MOST immediate cause of pain is probably 17.____

A. tissue damage
B. continuous stimulation
C. pressure in the cerebral cortex
D. excessive release of nerve energy
E. overstimulation

18. Typically, there is least hostility, most enjoyment, and most constructive work in groups where the leadership is 18.____

A. formal
B. laissez-faire
C. informal
D. autocratic
E. democratic

19. When people reproduce things from memory, a general characteristic is that remembered items are changed by 19.____

A. becoming less familiar in detail
B. omission of details
C. becoming less symmetrical
D. substitution of details
E. addition of details

20. The Young-Helmholtz theory of color vision holds that seeing the color yellow results from the simultaneous stimulation of ______ cones. 20.____

A. red and white
B. blue and red
C. blue and green
D. red and green
E. green and white

21. When ESP experiments have been done by different investigators under rigidly controlled conditions, the results 21.____

A. simply have not agreed
B. have been useless
C. prove conclusively that some people have extra-sensory perception
D. always have agreed
E. rule out ESP even as a possibility

22. A person interested in the study of the physiology of taste would also be interested in 22.____

A. tabes dorsalis
B. kinesthesis
C. alkaloids
D. papillae
E. free nerve endings

23. Generally, theories of color vision regard the eye as an instrument that 23.____

A. integrates and mixes effects of light
B. mixes light much as we mix colors in paint
C. has separate receptors for each hue
D. reflects light like a mirror
E. reduces light to its color elements

24. Rest periods should come at 24.____

A. mid-afternoon
B. immediately after production begins to drop
C. late morning
D. mid-morning
E. just before production falls off

25. The process of building up and breaking down stores of energy in the body is referred to as 25.____

A. homeostasis
B. hyperphaglia
C. ambiversion
D. opsin
E. metabolism

KEY (CORRECT ANSWERS)

1. C
2. D
3. B
4. A
5. B
6. E
7. C
8. E
9. B
10. E
11. C
12. D
13. B
14. D
15. B
16. B
17. A
18. E
19. B
20. D
21. A
22. D
23. A
24. E
25. E

TEST 3

DIRECTIONS: Each question or incomplete statement is followed by several suggested answers or completions. Select the one that BEST answers the question or completes the statement. *PRINT THE LETTER OF THE CORRECT ANSWER IN THE SPACE AT THE RIGHT.*

1. Any improvement in memory that occurs from memorizing nonsense syllables will be the result of 1.____

   A. exercise of the brain
   B. direct transfer
   C. reduced resistance to memorizing
   D. building of permanent neural connections for memory
   E. improved methods of memorizing

2. A primary group is one which is characterized by 2.____

   A. lack of prejudice
   B. democratic procedures
   C. natural leadership
   D. concern for people
   E. face-to-face relationships

3. In psychoanalysis, the importance of dreams lies in their 3.____

   A. continuity of content
   B. variety of content
   C. latent content
   D. freedom of expression
   E. manifest content

4. When events occur together in space and/or time, they are said to be 4.____

   A. antithetical
   B. contiguous
   C. conflicting
   D. identical
   E. conditioned

5. A psychotherapist whose patient has an extreme fear of parties arranges to get the patient to attend a party where he suffers no embarrassment and really likes and enjoys the party. 5.____
   This type of therapy is called

   A. supportive
   B. desensitization
   C. insight
   D. re-education
   E. hypnotic

6. At full maturity, Bill's height was only forty-six inches. Of the following glands, the one which was MOST likely involved in causing Bill's lack of growth is. 6.____

   A. gonads
   B. pituitary
   C. thyroid
   D. pancreas
   E. parathyroid

7. The development of irrational fears (phobias) in people is an illustration of 7.____

   A. extinction
   B. stimulus generalization
   C. partial reinforcement
   D. reinforcement
   E. instrumental learning

8. When two sets of measures (two factors) correlate highly, this means that 8.____

A. scores on the two factors will be in the same rank order
B. the two factors tend to vary together
C. scores will be the same on both factors
D. one factor causes the other
E. none of the above

9. Spearman found that the different parts of tests used to measure intelligence are inter-correlated. He concluded that this common element is basic to the total intellectual functioning of the individual. 9.____
He called this element

A. basic aptitude
B. *g*
C. intelligence
D. reasoning potential
E. *s*

10. The inborn aspect of intelligence is BEST represented by the term 10.____

A. flexibility
B. ability
C. versatility
D. adaptation
E. capacity

11. If we are trying to predict success or failure after training in a specific line of work, we would MOST likely administer a test of 11.____

A. aptitude
B. achievement
C. intelligence
D. personality
E. interest

12. The psychoanalytic process by which the patient regards the therapist in the same emotional context as he regarded his father is known as 12.____

A. contemporary causation
B. resistance
C. free association
D. functional autonomy
E. transference

13. Emotions are MOST closely similar to 13.____

A. perceptions
B. aspirations
C. images
D. habits
E. drives

14. The LOWEST type of feeblemindedness is known as 14.____

A. low normal
B. imbecile
C. idiot
D. borderline
E. moron

15. The MOST generally accepted explanation of forgetting is that it results from 15.____

A. conscious repression
B. interference by new learnings
C. inadequate original learning
D. reduced motivation
E. the passing of time

16. The central nervous system is located 16.____

A. within the skull and spinal column
B. near the surface of the body
C. in ganglion centers

D. only within the spinal column
E. within the whole body excluding extremities

17. The Thematic Apperception Test is made up of a series of 17.____

A. situational events
B. cartoons with the captions left off
C. geometric forms
D. ambiguous pictures
E. ink blots on a white background

18. Since fear motivates behavior, it must be considered 18.____

A. a drive
B. always constructive
C. as always overly observable
D. a positive goal
E. a weak response

19. The area of study which has provided the MOST information on cultures is 19.____

A. physiology
B. dermatology
C. psychology
D. anthropology
E. sociology

20. Learning consists of relatively permanent changes in behavior that are the result of 20.____

A. spontaneous recovery
B. gradients
C. experience
D. maturation
E. inherited tendencies

21. The psychoanalytic technique which requires the patient to say whatever comes to his mind regardless of how irrelevant or objectionable it may seem is called 21.____

A. cathexis
B. dream analysis
C. transference
D. free association
E. catharsis

22. Present evaluation of psychosurgery is that 22.____

A. it causes too little change in emotional reactions
B. it should be employed more extensively
C. less drastic and more effective treatment methods are now available
D. its effects are too temporary
E. it is the best technique for treating schizophrenia

23. The study reporting the results of various combinations of time spent in recitation as contrasted with time spent in reading found the MOST rewarding combination of reading and recitation to be 23.____

A. 60 percent reading, 40 percent recitation
B. 40 percent reading, 60 percent recitation
C. 80 percent recitation, 20 percent reading
D. 30 percent recitation, 70 percent reading
E. 50-50 split

24. One of the CHIEF characteristics of functionalism as a system of psychology was its emphasis on 24.____

    A. the study of the subconscious
    B. learned rather than unlearned behavior
    C. the study of the total behavior and experience of an individual
    D. the study of animal behavior
    E. the study of mental content

25. When compared with extremely intelligent children, on the average, normal children are found to be 25.____

    A. taller and heavier
    B. better adjusted socially
    C. more stable emotionally
    D. physically weaker
    E. healthier

KEY (CORRECT ANSWERS)

1. E
2. E
3. C
4. B
5. C

6. B
7. B
8. B
9. B
10. E

11. A
12. E
13. E
14. C
15. B

16. A
17. D
18. A
19. D
20. C

21. D
22. C
23. C
24. C
25. D

TEST 4

DIRECTIONS: Each question or incomplete statement is followed by several suggested answers or completions. Select the one that BEST answers the question or completes the statement. *PRINT THE LETTER OF THE CORRECT ANSWER IN THE SPACE AT THE RIGHT.*

1. A situation in which an organism slowly becomes accustomed to a fear-invoking stimulus and acts less and less frightened is known as 1.____

   A. habituation
   B. imprinting
   C. pseudo-conditioning
   D. inhibition
   E. sensitization

2. Vision is to retinal disparity as sound is to 2.____

   A. ear
   B. stereophonic
   C. eyeball
   D. facial vision
   E. brightness

3. The MAIN value of learning a general theory is that it helps one to 3.____

   A. demonstrate knowledge of a subject
   B. integrate a number of separate facts
   C. make mental associations
   D. express ideas easily
   E. avoid being specific

4. In a summary of several surveys, the MOST important item that workers said they wanted in a job was 4.____

   A. comfortable working conditions
   B. a good employer
   C. high pay
   D. opportunity for advancement
   E. job security

5. Hyperthyroidism causes 5.____

   A. mental deficiency
   B. sleepiness
   C. over-activity
   D. inactivity
   E. sluggishness

6. A detailed account of all the facts pertinent to a job is a 6.____

   A. employment table
   B. job analysis
   C. occupational index
   D. job list
   E. job description

7. The normal curve is an example of a 7.____

   A. pie chart
   B. histogram
   C. bar graph
   D. frequency polygon
   E. skewed distribution

8. The metabolic process is MOST dependent upon 8.____

   A. nitrogen
   B. hydrogen
   C. carbon dioxide
   D. oxygen
   E. carbon monoxide

9. Casual observation by a researcher led him to hypothesize that most drivers obey a certain traffic signal at an intersection. He then systematically observed traffic at the intersection in order to test his hypothesis. 9.____
   One may infer that the research was based on

   A. both inductive and deductive reasoning
   B. inductive reasoning
   C. deductive reasoning
   D. improper controls
   E. insufficient evidence

10. Experimental studies on transfer of training have caused psychologists to reject the principle of 10.____

   A. trial-and-error
   B. instrumental learning
   C. formal discipline
   D. S-R bonds
   E. negative transfer

11. Contiguity is especially relevant to 11.____

   A. size constancy
   B. the occurrence of two items closely together in time and place
   C. accommodation of the lens
   D. reduced cues
   E. perception

12. In the early days of psychotherapy, the MOST widely used technique was 12.____

   A. directive
   B. psychoanalytic
   C. client-centered
   D. non-directive
   E. eclectic

13. In evaluating the TAT and the Rorschach as measuring devices for personality characteristics, one may say correctly that they are 13.____

   A. nonverbal
   B. easily administered
   C. group tests
   D. objectively scored
   E. subtle kinds of interviews

14. If we were to learn the meaning of a word by hearing or seeing it used in different ways, we would have an example of concept formation by the method called 14.____

   A. definition
   B. context
   C. generalization
   D. classification
   E. discriminative learning

15. The term *equivalence of function* means that when a part of the brain is injured, very often the function of the damaged area 15.____

A. is completely lost to the animal
B. can be restored in the same area
C. is of so little importance it is not missed
D. appears as a malfunction in another brain area
E. is taken over by another area of the brain

16. Presenting the conditioning stimulus without reinforcement to an organism previously conditioned leads to 16.____

A. spontaneous discrimination
B. conditioned discrimination
C. extinction
D. spontaneous recovery
E. stimulus generalization

17. Studies which correlate the beliefs of a child with beliefs of parents show _______ correlation. 17.____

A. no positive
B. significant positive
C. no significant
D. low negative
E. perfect negative

18. Scientists have long been inclined to believe that the immediate stimulus for the sensation of pain is 18.____

A. overtaxing of cells
B. disturbed chemical balance
C. tissue injury
D. pressure
E. touching of certain nerve endings

19. The fact that the cerebral cortex is NOT functioning at birth means that 19.____

A. learning of complex behavior is delayed
B. the child will be developmentally retarded
C. all reflex behavior is impossible
D. crying is prevented
E. muscular movements cannot be made

20. A specialized psychotherapeutic technique designed to permit patients to act out roles, situations, and fantasies related to their problems is called 20.____

A. group therapy
B. play therapy
C. client-centered therapy
D. psychoanalysis
E. psychodrama

21. A person who is disturbed by groupings made of dots or dashes where some of the dots or dashes are missing is PROBABLY responding to the innate grouping factor called 21.____

A. illusion
B. proximity
C. similarity
D. continuation
E. symmetry

22. Aphasia means 22.____

A. loss of olfactory sensitivity
B. loss of ability to understand what is heard or read
C. word blindness
D. muscular incoordination
E. loss of memory

23. In psychoanalytic theory, that part of the personality conceived as a storehouse of motives and instinctual reactions is called the 23.____

A. sexual syndrome B. self C. ego
D. id E. superego

24. In psychoanalytic theory, that part of the personality which reconciles pleasure-seeking impulses with the reality of society is called the 24.____

A. libido B. ego C. conscience
D. superego E. id

25. The Bard-Cannon theory of emotions assumes that 25.____

A. all emotions are emergency reactions
B. feelings and bodily changes are simultaneously initiated through the hypothalamus
C. emotion is completely under intellectual control
D. feelings are the result of bodily changes
E. expressions of emotion are produced by feelings

KEY (CORRECT ANSWERS)

1. A
2. B
3. B
4. E
5. C

6. E
7. D
8. D
9. A
10. C

11. B
12. A
13. E
14. B
15. E

16. C
17. B
18. C
19. A
20. E

21. D
22. B
23. D
24. B
25. B

TEST 5

DIRECTIONS: Each question or incomplete statement is followed by several suggested answers or completions. Select the one that BEST answers the question or completes the statement. *PRINT THE LETTER OF THE CORRECT ANSWER IN THE SPACE AT THE RIGHT.*

1. If one were to punish an individual who is expressing anger, we could expect that person's level of anger to 1.____

   A. increase
   B. fluctuate in an unpredictable way
   C. drop to zero
   D. decrease
   E. remain relatively the same

2. Tranquilizers have the general characteristics of 2.____

   A. giving intellectual vigor
   B. keeping one awake in emergency situations
   C. reducing anxiety
   D. giving athletes more energy
   E. making one feel exhilarated

3. Gestalt psychology is characterized by 3.____

   A. analysis of sensations
   B. free association
   C. organization and configurations
   D. the study of conditioned reflexes
   E. an emphasis on introspection as in structuralism

4. Personal maladjustment is MOST likely to occur when the perceived self is 4.____

   A. radically different from the real self
   B. the individual's awareness of his own personality
   C. the result of past experiences
   D. traced to early infancy
   E. greatly influenced by learning

5. The research finding that the intelligence of fraternal twins correlates significantly HIGHER than that of sibling pairs indicates that 5.____

   A. fraternal twins are more intelligent than siblings
   B. environment is a factor
   C. heredity is a factor
   D. intelligence measures are unreliable
   E. siblings are more intelligent than fraternal twins

6. A reflex is 6.____

   A. exemplified in a recurrent nerve circuit
   B. an unlearned response to a stimulus
   C. the same as reaction time

D. the same as an instinct
E. any rapid response

7. An attribute is 7.____

A. unrelated to the physical aspects of a stimulus
B. in the stimulus rather than the observer
C. the total quality of a stimulus
D. a perceived aspect of a stimulus
E. exemplified by a tone

8. Sexual perversions are the result of 8.____

A. inadequate physical development
B. learning
C. lack of appropriate hormones
D. instinctive patterning
E. overly strong sex drive

9. At the synapse, 9.____

A. nerve impulses may reverse direction and travel back through the excited neuron
B. the nerve impulse from one neuron initiates an impulse in the adjoining neuron
C. direct neural connection is made with the spinal cord
D. nerve impulses pass from one neuron to the next
E. there is speeding up of the nerve impulse

10. Research tends to support the conclusion that thirst is the result of 10.____

A. cycling by action of the kidneys
B. loss of salt through sweating
C. dehydration of body cells
D. dryness of the mouth and throat
E. a shortage of water in the stomach

11. A probability of .01 would indicate that the obtained difference could be expected to occur by chance only once in _______ times. 11.____

A. 10 B. 100 C. 1,000 D. 10,000 E. 100,000

12. Differences in reaction time are MOST dependent upon the 12.____

A. diameter of the nerves involved
B. length of the nerves involved
C. number of synapses involved
D. amount of nerve energy involved
E. age of the person

13. Children in a family tend to have the same attitudes and beliefs as their parents because of 13.____

A. family loyalty
B. socio-economic status
C. discipline
D. hereditary factors
E. learning

14. A differential threshold should also be recognized as 14.____

    A. a just noticeable difference
    B. a proportion
    C. maximal discrimination
    D. a ratio
    E. a constant

15. If one child is 8 and another is 10 and both have an I.Q. of 120, the 10-year-old child is 15.____

    A. a near genius
    B. of the same intelligence as the 8 year old
    C. less intelligent
    D. brighter
    E. higher in mental age

16. The one essential for problem solving by the insight method is 16.____

    A. rote learning
    B. previous experience
    C. ability to use language
    D. to be over 12 years of age
    E. formal schooling

17. A trait is any aspect of personality that is 17.____

    A. easily observable but not necessarily quantifiable
    B. reasonably characteristic and distinctive
    C. observable and quantifiable on a ratio scale
    D. overt as well as covert
    E. factorially impure

18. With reference to interpretation of sex differences, research evidence shows that 18.____

    A. average differences between groups are small compared to differences within groups
    B. most intelligence tests discriminate against girls and in favor of boys
    C. girls are superior to boys in overall intelligence
    D. variability is not a factor when comparisons are made between groups
    E. boys are superior to girls in overall intelligence

19. A concept is generally learned more easily if it is 19.____

    A. pictured B. concrete C. abstract
    D. printed E. new

20. The scatter diagram for a correlation coefficient of +1.00 can be described BEST as 20.____

    A. either a straight line or a circle
    B. either an ellipse or a straight line
    C. a straight line
    D. elliptical
    E. circular

21. Variations in expressions of emotions are MOST evident in 21.____

A. chimpanzees
B. the Japanese
C. human children
D. human adults
E. monkeys

22. The median should be recognized as the 22.____

A. 25th percentile
B. 75th percentile
C. score that cuts a distribution in half
D. average
E. most frequently occurring score in a distribution

23. The organic psychosis which sometimes occurs as the result of syphilitic infection is known as 23.____

A. dementia praecox
B. neurasthenia
C. asphasia
D. general paresis
E. apraxia

24. If the items of a test are too difficult for the students taking it, a plotted curve of the distribution of the scores would be 24.____

A. rectangular
B. normal
C. bulged up in the center
D. skewed positively
E. skewed negatively

25. Unconscious problem solving is often assumed to take place during 25.____

A. trial-and-error
B. illumination
C. incubation
D. hypnosis
E. preparation

KEY (CORRECT ANSWERS)

1. A
2. C
3. C
4. A
5. B

6. B
7. D
8. B
9. B
10. C

11. B
12. C
13. E
14. A
15. E

16. B
17. B
18. A
19. B
20. C

21. D
22. C
23. D
24. D
25. C

EXAMINATION SECTION
TEST 1

DIRECTIONS: Each question or incomplete statement is followed by several suggested answers or completions. Select the one that BEST answers the question or completes the statement. *PRINT THE LETTER OF THE CORRECT ANSWER IN THE SPACE AT THE RIGHT.*

1. Which early approach in psychology fostered the development of modern-day applied psychology? 1.____

   A. Structuralism
   B. Behaviorism
   C. Functionalism
   D. Pragmatism

2. Psychology's answer to the question of whether we are *born* or *made* tends to be 2.____

   A. we are *born*
   B. we are *made*
   C. we are both *born* and *made*
   D. neither

3. With which of the following would a behaviorist agree? 3.____

   A. Conscious experiences can be studied in an objective, precise way.
   B. In order to understand behavior, one must understand the motives behind the behavior.
   C. Behavior can only be explained in terms of phenomenology, that is, an individual's interpretation of experience.
   D. Psychology should be the science of behavior that can be observed by others.

4. Which of the following would NOT be expected of an experimental psychologist? To 4.____

   A. study the effects of reward on learning
   B. look at the relationship between sleep deprivation and task performance
   C. conduct psychotherapy
   D. determine the forces that motivate behavior

5. For which of the following is Wilhelm Wundt primarily known? The 5.____

   A. establishment of the first formal laboratory for research in psychology
   B. distinction between mind and body as two separate entities
   C. discovery of how signals are conducted along nerves in the body
   D. development of the first formal program for training in psychotherapy

6. Nature is to nurture as heredity is to 6.____

   A. the environment
   B. instincts
   C. genetics
   D. maturation

7. *Conscious experiences and perceptions are more than the sum of their parts.* This statement is the basic premise of 7.___

A. introspectionism
B. structuralism
C. psychoanalysis
D. Gestalt psychology

8. G. Stanley Hall is noteworthy in the history of psychology because he 8.___

A. established the first American research laboratory in psychology
B. launched America's first psychological journal
C. was the driving force behind the establishment of the American Psychological Association
D. all of the above

9. A psychologist whose major interest is in how behavior changes as a function of age would specialize in the study of 9.___

A. personality
B. development
C. psychometrics
D. cognition

10. The two disciplines from which psychology emerged were 10.___

A. sociology and philosophy
B. philosophy and physiology
C. physiology and theology
D. physiology and sociology

11. Another name for the behavioral approach in psychology is 11.___

A. stimulus-response psychology
B. structuralism
C. applied psychology
D. Gestalt psychology

12. Janet trained her dog to sit on command by following this behavior with a reward of a dog biscuit and praise. Janet used the principles of 12.___

A. behaviorism
B. humanism
C. cognitive psychology
D. functionalism

13. Empiricism means that knowledge should be acquired through 13.___

A. logical reasoning
B. common sense
C. historical tradition
D. direct observation

14. According to Sigmund Freud, an individual's personality is largely determined by 14.___

A. self-actualizing tendencies
B. forces in the environment
C. strivings for superiority
D. forces in the unconscious

15. Humanists believe that people's behavior is governed by 15.___

A. their self-concepts
B. unconscious sexual urges
C. the outcomes of their responses
D. biochemical processes

16. The main contribution of physiology to the eventual emergence of psychology as a discipline was its 16.____

 A. emphasis on pure reasoning as the path to knowledge
 B. focus on body chemistry as the primary determinant of behavior
 C. emphasis on the scientific method as the primary means of collection information about behavior
 D. treatment of the mind and the body as two distinctly different entities

17. Which psychologist took the stand that organisms tend to repeat responses that lead to positive outcomes and tend not to repeat responses that lead to neutral or negative outcomes? 17.____

 A. Sigmund Freud B. B.F. Skinner
 C. Carl Rogers D. Abraham Maslow

18. Which early approach in psychology concentrated on breaking down conscious experience into its basic elements? 18.____

 A. Structuralism B. Behaviorism
 C. Functionalism D. Humanism

19. Which of the following demonstrates that psychology has evolved within a sociohistorical context? 19.____
The

 A. fact that Freud's theory of unconscious sexual conflicts developed during an era of repressed sexuality
 B. demand for psychological services during and after World War II
 C. rise of behaviorism in a pragmatic United States
 D. all of the above

20. B.F. Skinner's contention that behavior is fully determined by one's environment implies that 20.____

 A. we cannot really be held responsible for our actions
 B. punishment is the most effective method for controlling offensive behavior
 C. behavior is a function of genetic predispositions that are only minimally influenced by experience
 D. our thoughts and feelings are the result of reinforcement

21. It would be possible to have more than one ______ in a single data set. 21.____

 A. mean B. median
 C. mode D. none of the above

22. A hypothesis is a 22.____

 A. random guess as to what might happen in an experiment
 B. tentative statement about the relationship between two or more variables
 C. conclusion drawn from an experiment
 D. all of the above

23. Which of the following statements is FALSE? 23.___

    A. Psychologists sometimes expose animals to treatments that would be unacceptable with human subjects.
    B. There are absolutely no ethical restrictions on what can be done to animals in the name of science
    C. Only a small percentage of psychological studies involve animals.
    D. None of the above

24. The FINAL step in a scientific investigation is to 24.___

    A. conduct the study
    B. analyze the data
    C. decide whether or not the hypothesis was supported
    D. report the findings

25. A correlation coefficient of zero describes a ______ relationship between two variables. 25.___

    A. positive B. negative C. perfect D. lack of

KEY (CORRECT ANSWERS)

1. C	11. A
2. C	12. A
3. D	13. D
4. C	14. D
5. A	15. A
6. A	16. C
7. D	17. B
8. D	18. A
9. B	19. D
10. B	20. A

21. C
22. B
23. B
24. D
25. D

TEST 2

DIRECTIONS: Each question or incomplete statement is followed by several suggested answers or completions. Select the one that BEST answers the question or completes the statement. *PRINT THE LETTER OF THE CORRECT ANSWER IN THE SPACE AT THE RIGHT.*

1. A researcher wants to see if a protein-enriched diet will enhance the maze-running performance of rats. One group of rats is fed the high-protein diet for the duration of the study; the other group continues to receive ordinary rat chow. In this experiment, the diet fed to the two groups of rats is the ______ variable. 1.____

   A. correlated B. control C. dependent D. independent

2. In a study of personality and depression, Professor Norton finds a correlation of -.59 between optimism and depression and a correlation of .32 between introversion and depression. What can Professor Norton safely conclude? 2.____
   I. Optimism is inversely related to depression.
   II. Optimism is more strongly related to depression than is introversion.
   III. High optimism scores tend to be associated with low depression scores.
   IV. Low optimism causes high depression.

   The CORRECT answer is:

   A. I *only* B. II *only* C. I, II D. I, II, III E. I, II, III, IV

3. A psychologist monitors a group of nursery school children, recording each instance of altruistic behavior as it occurs. The psychologist is using 3.____

   A. the experimental method
   B. naturalistic observation
   C. case studies
   D. the survey method

4. The first step in a scientific investigation is to 4.____

   A. choose the subjects
   B. formulate a testable hypothesis
   C. choose a research method
   D. operationally define the variables

5. A researcher has children watch 30 minutes of violent television, and then counts the number of times they hit each other in a one-hour play period afterward as a measure of aggression. The researcher concludes that television violence causes aggression. However, this conclusion is invalid because 5.____

   A. there was no control group
   B. the study is strictly correlational
   C. aggression wasn't operationally defined
   D. it is unethical to force children to watch violent television

6. Researchers must describe the actions that will be taken to measure or control each variable in their studies. 6.____
   In other words, they must

   A. provide operational definitions of their variables
   B. decide if their studies will be experimental or correlational
   C. use statistics to summarize their findings
   D. decide how many subjects should participate in their studies

7. Which of the following correlation coefficients would indicate the STRONGEST relationship between two variables? 7.___

A. .58 B. .19 C. -.97 D. -.05

8. The experiment is a research method in which the investigator 8.___

A. systematically observes two variables to see whether there is an association between them
B. observes behavior as it occurs in its natural environment
C. conducts an in-depth investigation of an individual subject
D. manipulates a variable under carefully controlled conditions and observes whether there are changes in a second variable as a result

9. In the double-blind procedure, 9.___

A. subjects are unaware of which treatment condition they are in
B. the experimenter doesn't know which subjects are in the experimental or control groups
C. no one keeps track of who is in which group
D. both A and B

10. Random assignment of subjects occurs when 10.___

A. subjects are allowed to choose which group or condition in the study they would like to be in
B. a different method is used to assign each subject to a group or condition in the study
C. all subjects have an equal chance of being assigned to any group or condition in the study
D. all topics have an equal chance of being assigned to a particular experimenter

11. By definition, the population 11.___

A. is that group of people to whom the conclusion of the study will apply
B. is a subset of the sample
C. consists of those individuals who actually participate in the study
D. both A and B

12. Subjects' self-reports often indicate that they are healthier, happier, and less prejudiced than other types of evidence would suggest. The MOST likely explanation is 12.___

A. experimenter bias
B. faulty memory
C. the social desirability bias
D. a tendency to agree with almost every statement

13. Any measurable conditions, events, characteristics, or behaviors that are controlled or observed in a study are called 13.___

A. hypotheses B. correlations
C. variables D. confounds

14. The standard deviation is a measure of 14.____

A. central tendency
B. the amount of variability in a data set
C. the degree of relationship between two variables
D. the difference between the largest and smallest scores in a data set

15. In an experiment, the variable that is ultimately measured is called the ______ variable. 15.____

A. dependent
B. independent
C. observed
D. response

16. Suppose that high alcohol consumption among college students is associated with low grade point averages. Based on this information, we can conclude that 16.____

A. high alcohol consumption causes students to get lower grades
B. getting low grades causes students to drink more alcohol
C. stress causes students both to get lower grades and to consume more alcohol
D. none of the above

17. Experimenter bias occurs when 17.____

A. experimenters' beliefs in their own hypotheses affect either the subjects' behavior or their observations of the subjects
B. experimenters explicitly instruct the subjects to behave in a way that will be consistent with the hypothesis
C. experimenters desire to make a favorable impression on their subjects
D. experimenters conduct their studies in a completely objective manner

18. The correlation coefficient is a measure of 18.____

A. central tendency
B. the amount of variability in a data set
C. the degree of relationship between two variables
D. the difference between the largest and smallest scores in a data set

19. The independent variable is a hypothesized ______; the dependent variable is a hypothesized ______. 19.____

A. cause; cause
B. cause; effect
C. effect; effect
D. effect; cause

20. Suppose that students who work more hours at their jobs tend to have lower grade point averages, and that they also tend to get less sleep. If we were to correlate the two variables of grade point average and number of hours at work, we would find ______ relationship. 20.____

A. no
B. a positive
C. a negative

21. When psychologists say that their results are statistically significant, they mean that the results 21.___

    A. have important practical applications
    B. have important implications for scientific theory
    C. are unlikely to be due to the fluctuations of chance
    D. all of the above

22. A confounding of variables occurs when 22.___

    A. two or more variables are linked together in a way that makes it difficult to sort out their specific effects
    B. the sample is not representative of the population
    C. subjects are influenced by the social desirability bias
    D. subjects experience some change from a nonexistent or ineffective treatment due to their expectations

23. By definition, a sample 23.___

    A. is that group of people to whom the conclusion of the study will apply
    B. is a subset of the population
    C. consists of those individuals who actually participate in the study
    D. both B and C

24. In descriptive/correlational research, the investigator 24.___

    A. systematically observes two variables to see whether there is an association between them
    B. manipulates a variable under carefully controlled conditions and observes whether there are changes in a second variable as a result
    C. exposes subjects to two closely related treatment conditions
    D. manipulates two or more independent variables simultaneously

25. Replication involves 25.___

    A. having each subject participate in the experiment several times to check the accuracy of the results
    B. manipulating several independent variables at once
    C. having each subject participate in both the experimental and control groups
    D. the repetition of a study to see whether the earlier results are duplicated

KEY (CORRECT ANSWERS)

1. D
2. D
3. B
4. B
5. A

6. A
7. C
8. D
9. D
10. C

11. A
12. C
13. C
14. B
15. A

16. D
17. A
18. C
19. B
20. C

21. C
22. A
23. D
24. A
25. D

TEST 3

DIRECTIONS: Each question or incomplete statement is followed by several suggested answers or completions. Select the one that BEST answers the question or completes the statement. *PRINT THE LETTER OF THE CORRECT ANSWER IN THE SPACE AT THE RIGHT.*

1. Internal functions such as heartbeat, breathing, and stomach contractions are controlled by the _______ nervous system. 1.____

   A. central B. autonomic C. somatic D. endocrine

2. When a dominant gene is paired with a recessive gene, the gene pair is said to be 2.____

   A. homozygous B. phenotypic
   C. heterozygous D. polygenic

3. Damage to the cerebellum is MOST likely to result in 3.____

   A. problems with coordination of movement
   B. impairment of short-term memory
   C. difficulties in judging distance
   D. eating irregularities

4. A marathon runner may well experience a phenomenon known as *runner's high* because the pain of a long run may trigger the release of _______ in the brain. 4.____

   A. morphine B. endorphins
   C. placebos D. naloxone

5. The master gland of the endocrine system is the 5.____

   A. thyroid gland B. adrenal gland
   C. pancreas D. pituitary gland

6. The basic parts of a neuron are 6.____

   A. vesicles, terminal buttons, synapse
   B. cell body, axon, dendrites
   C. myelin, nodes, axon terminals
   D. hindbrain, midbrain, forebrain

7. A person might end up in a coma if the following area of the brain is damaged: 7.____

   A. Reticular formation B. Medulla
   C. Hypothalamus D. Pons

8. _______ function in the endocrine system much like _______ in the nervous system. 8.____

   A. Hormones; dendrites
   B. Hormones; neurotransmitters
   C. Endorphins; sensory neurons
   D. Neurotransmitters; hormones

9. Which of the following structures is not part of the hindbrain? 9.____

   A. Cerebellum B. Thalamus
   C. Medulla D. Pons

10. An inadequate supply of ______ in the brain has been implicated as a factor in the memory loss seen with Alzheimer's disease. 10.____

A. dopamine
B. acetylcholine
C. serotonin
D. norepinephrine

11. When one member of a gene pair is more influential, such that its trait is expressed over the trait of the other gene, it is said to be 11.____

A. expressive
B. genotypic
C. phenotypic
D. dominant

12. The ______ is the junction between two neurons. 12.____

A. synapse
B. terminal button
C. postsynaptic membrane
D. node

13. Research results indicate that lefthanders are over-represented in groups suffering from all but which of the following? 13.____

A. Alcoholism
B. Schizophrenia
C. Mental retardation
D. Multiple personality disorder

14. A neural impulse is initiated when a neuron's charge momentarily becomes less negative, or even positive.
This event is called 14.____

A. an action potential
B. a resting potential
C. impulse facilitation
D. neuromodulation

15. In people whose corpus callosums have not been severed, verbal stimuli are identified more quickly and more accurately when 15.____

A. sent to the right hemisphere first
B. sent to the left hemisphere first
C. presented to the left visual field
D. presented auditorally rather than visually

16. The blood-brain barrier is a semipermeable membrane-like mechanism that 16.____

A. keeps neurotransmitters from entering the bloodstream
B. stops some chemicals from passing from the bloodstream to the brain
C. prevents ions in the blood from entering the brain
D. regulates the flow of blood to the brain and spinal cord

17. A split-brain person has a severed 17.____

A. cerebral cortex
B. cerebellum
C. medulla
D. corpus callosum

18. An impulse moves from one neuron to another through the action of 18.____

A. neurotransmitters
B. hormones
C. action potentials
D. neuromodulators

19. The ______ is the largest and most complex part of the human brain. 19.____

A. medulla
B. cerebrum
C. cerebellum
D. limbic system

20. The main reason for the characterization of the left hemisphere as the *dominant* hemisphere was 20.____

A. the evidence that the left hemisphere usually processes language
B. the evidence that the left hemisphere usually processes complex information
C. the fact that the majority of people are righthanded
D. that split-brain patients use only their left hemisphere for processing information

Questions 21-25.

DIRECTIONS: Questions 21 through 25 are to be answered on the basis of the brain chart shown below.

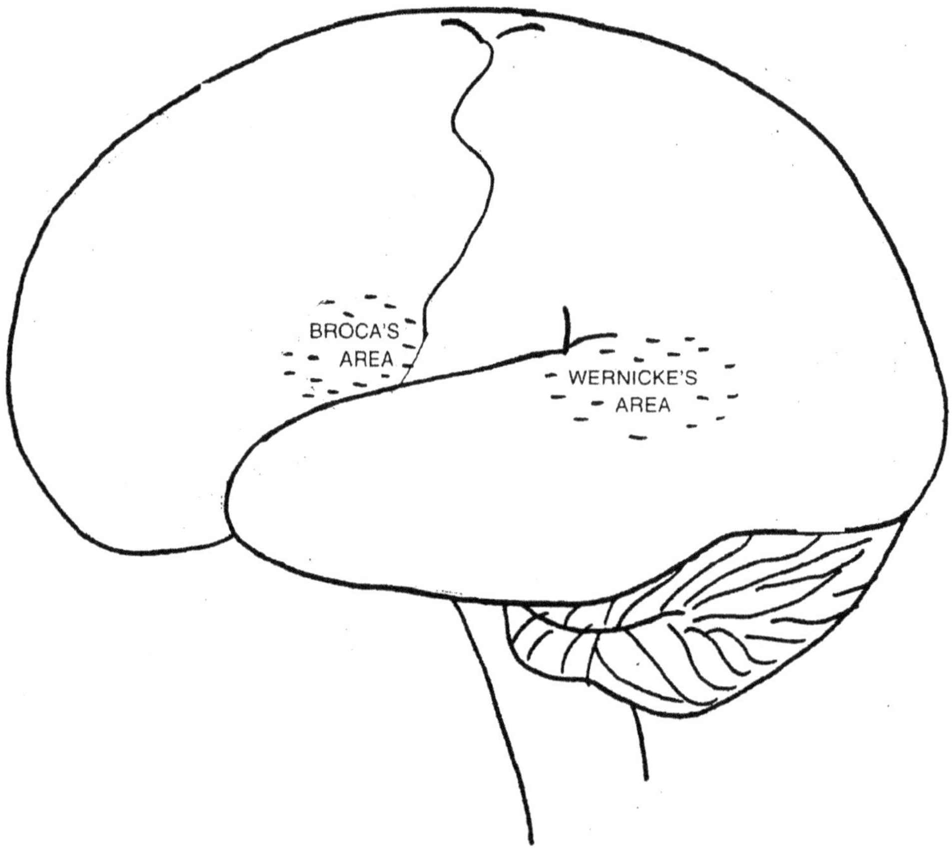

21. Identify and name the area that is responsible for handling visual information. 21.____

22. Identify the area responsible for higher mental processes, motor movement, planning, and impulse control. 22.____

23. Identify and name the area that is responsible for processing tactile information. 23.____

24. Identify and name the area that is responsible for processing of auditory information. 24.____

25. Circle the area that if lesioned will produce difficulties in the production of speech. 25.____

KEY (CORRECT ANSWERS)

1. B
2. C
3. A
4. B
5. D
6. B
7. A
8. B
9. B
10. B
11. A
12. A
13. D
14. A
15. B
16. B
17. D
18. A
19. B
20. A
21. Occipital lobe
22. Frontal lobe
23. Parietal lobe
24. Temporal lobe

EXAMINATION SECTION
TEST 1

DIRECTIONS: Each question or incomplete statement is followed by several suggested answers or completions. Select the one that BEST answers the question or completes the statement. *PRINT THE LETTER OF THE CORRECT ANSWER IN THE SPACE AT THE RIGHT.*

1. A recurrent bilateral conjunctivitis occurring with onset of hot weather with burning, itching and lacrimation with polygonal raised areas usually found in young boys is called 1.____

   A. trachoma
   B. phlyctenular conjunctivitis
   C. mucopurulent conjunctivitis
   D. vernal conjunctivitis

2. A patient using contact lenses develops a corneal infection. A diagnosis of acanthamoeba keratitis is established after laboratory investigations. The best drug for treatment is 2.____

   A. propamidine isothienate
   B. neosporine
   C. ketoconazole
   D. polyhexamethylene biguanide

3. SAFE strategy has been described for the control of 3.____

   A. onchocerciasis
   B. trachoma
   C. refractive error
   D. ocular trauma

4. Type IV hypersensitivity to mycobacterium tuberculosis antigen may clinically show as 4.____

   A. iridocyclitis
   B. phlyctenular conjunctivitis
   C. disciform keratitis
   D. deep keratitis

5. A 30-year-old male has a past injury to the eye with leaf followed by pain, photophobia and redness. What is the most likely pathology? 5.____

   A. Conjunctivitis
   B. Iridicyclitis
   C. Fungal corneal ulcer
   D. Corneal laceration

6. Which of the following is not needed to be present for clinical diagnosis of trachoma? 6.____

   A. Panus
   B. Follicles
   C. Papillae
   D. Superficial punctate keratitis

7. The normal human cornea 7.____

A. has refractive index more than air
B. is more than one millimeter thick
C. is innervated by terminal branches of supratrochlear nerve
D. receives most of its oxygen supply from limbal circulation

8. Conjunctival follicles are often found in 8.____

A. neonatal conjunctivitis caused by *chlamydia trachomatis*
B. adult conjunctivitis caused by *chlamydia trachomatis*
C. ocular cicatricial pemphigoid
D. Stevens Johnson syndrome

9. Neurotrophic kerotapathy 9.____

A. results from damage to the VII cranial nerve
B. may be associated with a persistent epithelial defect
C. is more likely with herpes simplex virus than with herpes zoster virus
D. produces decreased osmolarity of tear film

10. Which of the following statements regarding Vitamin A deficiency is incorrect? 10.____

A. Bitot spots are composed of keratin
B. Night blindness often precedes xerophthalmia
C. Vitamin deficiency can occur as a result of an intestinal malabsorption
D. Children with Vitamin A deficiency have fewer infections because of immune hyper-reactivity X

11. Which of the following statements is incorrect? 11.____

A. Fleischer ring is found in keratoconus and is an iron line around the base of cone
B. Stocker line is associated with pterygium
C. Ferry line is found in filtering bleb
D. Silver deposit within the cornea is called chysiasis

12. Stevens Johnson syndrome 12.____

A. is commonly associated with drug hypersensitivity
B. rarely presents with an acute febrile episode
C. is not associated with dry eye
D. is generally the disease of the young

13. Each of the following is associated with keratoconus EXCEPT 13.____

A. Down syndrome
B. retinitis pigmentosa
C. Marian's syndrome
D. tuberculosis

14. Soft contact lens users have very high tendency to develop 14.____

A. acanthamoeba ulcer
B. recurrent corneal ulcer

C. pseudomonas ulcer
D. trachoma

15. Recurrent corneal erosion is a feature of 15.____

A. keratoglobus
B. keratoconus
C. glaucoma
D. corneal dystrophy

16. Causes of childhood blindness include all of the following EXCEPT 16.____

A. measles
B. ophthalmia neonatorum
C. rubella
D. Vitamin B deficiency

17. An ocular symptom not seen in acute herpes zoster is 17.____

A. nummular keratitis
B. glaucoma
C. uveitis
D. cranial nerve palsy

18. An 11-year-old boy has experienced intense itching, foreign body sensation and ropy discharge during the last seven summer seasons. The most likely cause is 18.____

A. viral conjunctivitis
B. trachoma
C. vernal keratoconjunctivitis
D. acanthamoeba keratitis

19. A 40-year-old male complains of pain, redness and photophobia. What is the most probable diagnosis? 19.____

A. Chronic uveitis
B. Conjunctivitis
C. Keratitis
D. Blepharitis

20. Which of the following is not seen in iron pigmentation of the cornea? 20.____

A. Ferry's line
B. Stacker's line
C. Hudson-Stahli line
D. Krukenberg's spindle

21. In bullous keratopathy, there is damage to the 21.____

A. epithelium
B. stromal layer
C. endothelium
D. Descemet's membrane

22. Tear film is absent in 22.____

    A. surgical removal of lacrimal gland
    B. keratoconjunctivitis sicca
    C. herpes keratitis
    D. chronic uveitis

23. Salmon patch is seen in 23.____

    A. interstitial keratitis
    B. trachoma
    C. angular conjunctivitis
    D. phlyctenular keratitis

24. Ophthalmia neonatorum caused by gonococci manifest within 24.____

    A. hours
    B. 1-3 days
    C. 5-8 days
    D. 10-12 days

25. In photophthalmia, the treatment administered should be 25.____

    A. topical anesthetics
    B. steroid eye drops
    C. topical antibiotics
    D. eye pad

26. The complications of soft contact lenses include all of the following EXCEPT 26.____

    A. corneal abrasion
    B. allergic reaction
    C. infection
    D. retinal detachment

27. The organism which can penetrate intact corneal epithelium is 27.____

    A. streptococcus pyogenes
    B. staphylococcus epidermidis
    C. pseudomonas pyocyanaea
    D. corynebacterium diphtheriae

28. All of the following are features of keratoconus EXCEPT 28.____

    A. distorted corneal reflex
    B. myopic astigmatism
    C. increased corneal thickness
    D. Fleischer's ring

29. Angular conjunctivitis is usually caused by 29.____

    A. moraxella
    B. chlamydia trachomatis
    C. pneumococcus
    D. gonococcus

30. Arlt's line is present in 30.____

    A. upper palpebral conjunctiva
    B. lower palpebral conjunctiva
    C. bulbar conjunctiva
    D. sclera

31. All of the following are associated with trachoma EXCEPT 31.____

    A. follicular hypertrophy
    B. papillary hyperplasia
    C. Herbert's pits
    D. Horner-Trantas dots

32. Sequalae of trachoma include 32.____

    A. pseudoptosis
    B. cicatricial entropion
    C. trichiasis
    D. all of the above

33. All of the following statements regarding Mooren's ulcer are true EXCEPT 33.____

    A. it is a superficial ulcer starting at the corneal margin
    B. pain is absent
    C. it has an advancing border
    D. it is treated with topical steroids and immunosuppressives

34. The most common cause of ulcus serpens is 34.____

    A. pneumococcus
    B. gonococcus
    C. staphylococcus
    D. corynebacterium diphtheriae

35. Snow blindness is caused by 35.____

    A. vasoconstriction due to decreased temperature at high altitude
    B. acute papillitis due to cold
    C. photo-ophthalmia due to reflection of ultraviolet rays from the snow surface
    D. infrared rays

36. Band-shaped keratopathy is commonly caused by deposition of ______ salt. 36.____

    A. magnesium
    B. calcium
    C. ferrous
    D. zinc

37. Corneal sensations are lost in 37.____

    A. herpes simplex
    B. scleritis
    C. fungal infection
    D. angular conjunctivitis

38. Which of the following are features of herpes simplex keratitis? 38.____

A. Dendritic ulcer
B. Geographical ulcer
C. Disciform keratitis
D. All of the above

39. Deep leucomatous corneal opacity is best treated by 39.____

A. tattooing
B. lamellar keratoplasty
C. photorefractive keratectomy
D. all of the above

40. Hutchinson's sign is due to involvement of which cranial nerve? 40.____

A. Lacrimal
B. Nasociliary
C. Maxillary
D. Mandibular

41. Regarding interstitial keratitis, which of the following is false? 41.____

A. It is commonly seen in syphilis, tuberculosis and leprosy
B. It is an inflammation involving full thickness of cornea
C. Salmon patch is a pathognomic finding
D. Treatment involves topical steroids, cycloplegics and specific etiological treatment

42. Which stain is used specially for acanthamoeba keratitis? 42.____

A. Gram's
B. Giemsa's
C. Calcofluor white
D. Rose Bengal

43. A child has a congenital cataract involving the visual axis. It is detected when the child is 10 days old. The best time for surgery is 43.____

A. immediately
B. at 3 months of age
C. at 6 months of age
D. at 3 years of age

44. The length of corneal incision in phacoemulsification surgery is ______ mm. 44.____

A. 1 -1.5
B. 2-2.5
C. 3-3.5
D. 3.5-4.5

45. The normal, aging human crystalline lens 45.____

A. develops an increasingly curved shape, resulting in more refractive power
B. develops an increasingly flatter shape, resulting in less refractive power
C. undergoes an increase in index of refraction as a result of decreasing presence of insoluble protein particles
D. undergoes a decrease in index of refraction as a result of decreasing presence of insoluble protein particles

46. With accommodation, 46.____

A. most of the change in lens shape occurs in the central anterior capsule
B. most of the change in lens shape occurs in the peripheral anterior capsule
C. most of the change in lens shape occurs in the peripheral posterior capsule
D. lens shape changes are equally distributed throughout both anterior and posterior surfaces

47. Which of the following statements is incorrect? 47.____

A. Second sight is caused by lenticular myopia
B. Monocular diplopia caused by cataracts cannot be corrected with glasses
C. Mild posterior subcapsular cataracts do not cause visual symptoms
D. Cataracts can cause greater impairment in contrast sensitivity than in Snellen's acuity

48. The lens contains the oldest fibers in the 48.____

A. nucleus
B. nucleo-cortical junction
C. anterior surface
D. posterior surface

49. The associations of microspheropakia include all EXCEPT 49.____

A. Marfan's syndrome
B. retinoblastoma
C. hyperlysinaernia
D. Marchesani syndrome

50. The optimal time to treat a dense, bilateral cataract is 50.____

A. immediately
B. between two and six months
C. between six months and one year of age
D. between one and two years of age

KEY (CORRECT ANSWERS)

1. D	11. D	21. C	31. D	41. B
2. D	12. A	22. B	32. D	42. C
3. B	13. D	23. A	33. B	43. A
4. C	14. C	24. C	34. A	44. C
5. C	15. D	25. D	35. C	45. A
6. D	16. D	26. D	36. B	46. A
7. A	17. B	27. D	37. A	47. C
8. B	18. C	28. C	38. D	48. A
9. B	19. C	29. A	39. D	49. B
10. D	20. D	30. A	40. B	50. A

TEST 2

DIRECTIONS: Each question or incomplete statement is followed by several suggested answers or completions. Select the one that BEST answers the question or completes the statement. *PRINT THE LETTER OF THE CORRECT ANSWER IN THE SPACE AT THE RIGHT.*

1. After enucleation of the eyeball, a properly sized artificial prosthetic eye is advisable after a post-operative period of 1.____

   A. about 14 days
   B. about 20 days
   C. 6-8 weeks
   D. 12-24 weeks

2. Bilateral ptosis is seen in 2.____

   A. trauma
   B. Marfan's syndrome
   C. myasthenia gravis
   D. tumors

3. A 30-year-old male has blunt trauma to the orbit with diplopia and enophthalmos. X-rays of the orbit reveals a blow out fracture. Which wall of the orbit is most likely fractured? 3.____

   A. Lateral
   B. Superior
   C. Medial
   D. Inferior

4. A 50-year-old female is experiencing difficulty swallowing food along with ptosis and diplopia when looking in all directions. What is the probable diagnosis? 4.____

   A. Lateral rectus palsy
   B. Oculomotor palsy
   C. Presbyopia
   D. Myasthenia gravis

5. An important sign of carotid cavernous fistula is 5.____

   A. intermittent proptosis
   B. pulsating proptosis
   C. Homer's syndrome
   D. enophthalmos

6. A patient is experiencing recurrent chalazion, and histopathology reveals carcinomatous changes. This condition is 6.____

   A. sebaceous cell carcinoma
   B. squamous cell carcinoma
   C. adenocarcinoma
   D. basal cell carcinoma

7. The clinical features of cavernous sinus thrombosis include all EXCEPT 7.____

   A. ophthalmoplegia
   B. swelling of mastoid region
   C. diminution of vision
   D. enophthalmos

8. Intermittent proptosis is seen in 8.____

   A. varicosity of ophthalmic vein
   B. cavernous sinus thrombosis
   C. carotid cavernous fistula
   D. severe thyrotoxicosis

9. The muscles which are involved earliest in thyroid ophthalmology are 9.____

   A. lateral rectus
   B. medial rectus
   C. inferior oblique
   D. superior rectus

10. All of the following clinical features may be present in a patient with facial nerve paralysis EXCEPT 10.____

   A. lower eyelid ectropion
   B. blepharospasm
   C. inability to close eyes
   D. epiphora

11. A 2-year-old child has a round, well-demarcated mass at the supero-temporal rim. The overlying skin is normal, and the lesion has been present since birth. The most likely diagnosis is 11.____

   A. rhabdomysarcoma
   B. neurofibroma
   C. dermoid cyst
   D. capillary hemangioma

12. Which of the following is the most common clinical feature of Graves' ophthalmopathy? 12.____

   A. Exophthalmos
   B. External ophthalmoplegia
   C. Eyelid retraction
   D. Optic neuropathy

13. The most common determinant in selecting a corrective procedure for any type of ptosis is 13.____

   A. vertical height of palpebral aperture
   B. age of patient
   C. amount of levator function
   D. duration of ptosis

14. The condition that is characterized by a drooping eyelid and wrinkled skin after repeated attacks of eyelid edema is called 14.____

   A. blepharoptosis
   B. blepharospasm
   C. blepharochalasis
   D. blepharophimosis

15. A 75-year-old woman complains of tearing and discharge upon pressing the medial canthus of her right eye. When syringing from the lower canaliculus, regurgitation of mucopurulent fluid takes place. The most appropriate treatment is 15.____

A. dacryocystorhinostomy
B. probing and syringing
C. antiglaucoma drugs
D. antibiotics

16. Everbusch's operation is indicated for 16.____

A. proptosis
B. ptosis
C. ectropion
D. entropion

17. Distichiasis is the ______ of eyelashes. 17.____

A. misdirection
B. accessory layer
C. absence
D. scarcity

18. Cicatricial entropion occurs secondary to all of these conditions EXCEPT 18.____

A. Cicatricial pemphigoid
B. trachoma
C. corneal ulcer
D. chemical burns

19. Modified Kuhnt Szymanowski procedure is done for 19.____

A. ectropion
B. entropion
C. dermoid
D. ptosis

20. All of the following are features of canaliculitis EXCEPT 20.____

A. frequently caused by Actinomyces israelii
B. characterized by pouting punctum and concretions within the canaliculus
C. treatment is canaliculotomy
D. possible swelling in lacrimal sac region

21. Treatment of choice for ptosis with Marcus Gunn jaw winking phenomenon is 21.____

A. LPS resection
B. skin excision
C. unilateral frontalis sling operation
D. bilateral frontalis sling operation

22. Congenital ptosis is a type of ______ ptosis. 22.____

A. myogenic
B. neurogenic
C. traumatic
D. synkinetic

23. A 9-month-old male child has epiphora, blepharospasm and photophobia. The probable diagnosis is 23.____

A. congenital cataract
B. anterior uveitis
C. congenital glaucoma
D. retinal detachment

24. Tonography helps us determine 24.____

A. rate of formation of aqueous
B. the facility of outflow of aqueous
C. the levels of IOP at different times
D. field changes

25. Which one of these clinical features would be helpful in the diagnosis of open angle glaucoma? 25.____

A. Cupping of optic disc
B. Depth of anterior chamber
C. Visual acuity
D. Angle of anterior chamber

26. The drug of choice for acute angle closure glaucoma is 26.____

A. 2% pilocarpine
B. timolol
C. dorzolamide
D. atropine

27. The most common senile cataract causing glaucoma is 27.____

A. incipient type
B. nuclear type
C. morgagnian type
D. sclerotic hypermature

28. All of the following features are associated with primary angle closure glaucoma EXCEPT 28.____

A. small cornea
B. keratoglobus
C. shallow anterior chamber
D. short axial length of eyeball

29. Rubeosis iridis is most commonly caused by 29.____

A. diabetes mellitus
B. Eale's disease
C. retinoblastoma
D. retinal detachment

30. History of colored haloes is present in all of the following EXCEPT 30.____

A. mucopurulent conjunctivitis
B. angle closure glaucoma
C. uveitis
D. corneal edema

31. Increased intraocular pressure is seen in all of the following EXCEPT 31.____

A. epidemic dropsy
B. branch retinal vein occlusion
C. malignant melanoma
D. phthisis bulbi

32. The earliest field defect in primary open angle glaucoma is 32.____

A. Seidel's scotoma
B. arcuate scotoma
C. nasal step
D. paracentral scotoma

33. The trabeculodysgenesis is part of the pathophysiology of the following glaucomas EXCEPT 33.____

A. Sturge-Weber syndrome
B. homocystinuria
C. aniridia
D. Peters Anomaly

34. In the instance of an irregular cornea, the best type of tonometer to use is 34.____

A. applanation
B. Schiotz
C. handheld applanation
D. Mackay-Marg

35. The applanation tonometer is based on ______ law. 35.____

A. Lincoff's
B. Stake's
C. Imbert-Fick's
D. Boyle's

36. The treatment of choice for phacomorphic glaucoma is 36.____

A. paracentesis from anterior chamber
B. lens extraction
C. medical treatment of glaucoma
D. trabeculectomy

37. Inheritance of congenital glaucoma is 37.____

A. autosomal dominant
B. autosomal recessive
C. X-linked recessive
D. none of the above

38. Early clinical features of congenital glaucoma include all of the following EXCEPT 38.____

A. epiphora
B. photophobia
C. corneal enlargement
D. corneal edema

39. Angle recession glaucoma presents as 39.____

A. acute rise of IOP
B. chronic rise of IOP
C. biphasic presentation
D. none of the above

40. Normal cup size in the optic disc is 40.____

A. 0.1 to 0.2
B. 0.2 to 0.3
C. 0.3 to 0.4
D. 0.5 to 0.6

41. The main site of obstruction in primary open angle glaucoma is 41.____

A. at Schlemm's canal
B. juxtacanalicular trabecular meshwork
C. episcleral veins
D. scleral channels

42. All of the following are seen in the optic nerve head in a case of OAG EXCEPT 42.____

A. splinter hemorrhage
B. fullness of optic cup
C. bayoneting sign
D. baring of circumlinear vessels

43. A soldier complains of difficulty in reading the newspaper with his right eye four weeks after sustaining a gunshot injury to his left eye. The most likely diagnosis is 43.____

A. retinal detachment
B. sympathetic ophthalmitis
C. traumatic avulsion of optic nerve
D. delayed vitreous hemorrhage

44. In a patient with AIDS, chorioretinitis is typically caused by 44.____

A. cytomegalovirus
B. toxoplasma gondii
C. toxocara
D. cryptococcus neoformans

45. Uveitis is seen in 45.____

A. ankylosing spondylitis
B. psoriasis
C. Marian's syndrome
D. lichen planus

46. All of the following features are correct in regards to heterochromic iridocyclitis of Fuchs EXCEPT 46.____

A. hyperpigmented iris
B. hypopigmented iris
C. coarse keratic precipitates
D. glaucoma

47. Of the following statements, which is NOT true regarding sympathetic ophthalmitis? 47.____

A. It is more common after perforating injury in the ciliary body region
B. It is more common if suppuration takes place in the exciting eye
C. Begins 4-6 weeks after injury
D. Injury to the opposite eye is the preceding event

48. Toxoplasma usually affects the 48.____

A. macula
B. iris
C. ciliary body
D. oraserrata

49. Which of these patients with juvenile rheumatoid arthritis is at highest risk of developing ocular complications? 49.____

A. A 5-year-old boy with fever, rash, lymphadenopathy and arthritis of the ankle with negative ANA result
B. A 3-year-old boy with arthritis of the hands, wrist, ankle and knee, a positive ANA result and positive rheumatoid factor
C. A 2-year-old girl with mild arthritis of the left knee and ankle, a positive ANA result and a negative rheumatoid factor
D. A 10-year-old boy with arthritis of the hip girdle, negative ANA result and negative rheumatoid factor

50. Treatment for ocular toxoplasmosis includes all of the following EXCEPT 50.____

A. sulphonamides
B. clindamycin
C. pyrimethamine
D. periocular steroids

KEY (CORRECT ANSWERS)

1. C	11. C	21. D	31. D	41. B
2. C	12. C	22. A	32. D	42. B
3. D	13. C	23. C	33. B	43. B
4. D	14. C	24. B	34. D	44. A
5. B	15. A	25. C	35. C	45. A
6. A	16. B	26. A	36. B	46. C
7. D	17. B	27. C	37. B	47. B
8. A	18. B	28. B	38. C	48. A
9. B	19. A	29. A	39. C	49. C
10. B	20. D	30. C	40. C	50. D

TEST 3

DIRECTIONS: Each question or incomplete statement is followed by several suggested answers or completions. Select the one that BEST answers the question or completes the statement. *PRINT THE LETTER OF THE CORRECT ANSWER IN THE SPACE AT THE RIGHT.*

1. Which of the following statements about sympathetic ophthalmitis is true? 1.____

   A. It occurs only after penetrating injury with uveal prolapse
   B. It may occur as early as ten days or as late as 50 years following the suspected triggering incident
   C. It is characterized by intense lymphocytic infitration in the choroids and choriocapillaries
   D. Dalen-Fuchs nodules are pathognomic findings of sympathetic ophthalmia

2. All of the following are part of the uvea EXCEPT 2.____

   A. pars plicata
   B. pars plana
   C. choroids
   D. Schwalbe's line

3. All of the following are typical clinical features of uveitis EXCEPT 3.____

   A. Pain
   B. Ciliary congestion
   C. Mucopurulent discharge
   D. Small pupil

4. Typical coloboma of the iris is situated 4.____

   A. nasally
   B. inferonasally
   C. temporally
   D. inferotemporally

5. A sign of acuity in the uveitis is 5.____

   A. aqueous flare
   B. cells in the anterior chamber
   C. constricted pupil
   D. raised intraocular pressure

6. A child with healed central choroiditis in one or both eyes should be investigated for 6.____

   A. histoplasmosis
   B. toxoplasmosis
   C. entamoeba histolytica
   D. tuberculosis

7. Sjogren's syndrome consists of all of these features EXCEPT 7.____

   A. keratoconjunctivitis sicca
   B. xerostomia with or without salivary gland enlargement
   C. seropositive rheumatoid arthritis
   D. interstitial keratitis

8. Which of the following syndromes consist of symmetrical enlargement of salivary and lacrimal glands? 8.____

   A. Sjogren's
   B. Mikulicz's
   C. Sturge-Weber
   D. Vogt Koyonagi Harada

9. Causes of scleritis include all of the following EXCEPT 9.____

   A. herpes zoster
   B. rheumatoid arthritis
   C. trachoma
   D. tuberculosis

10. All of the following statements regarding anterior necrotizing scleritis with inflammation are true EXCEPT 10.____

   A. it is a very severe form of scleritis with pain and redness
   B. avascular patches may be present in the sclera
   C. there may be associated anterior uveitis
   D. treatment includes nonsteroidal anti-inflammatory drugs

11. A vitreous aspirate is collected from a patient with endophthalmitis in eye casualty. Regarding storage, the sample should be 11.____

   A. kept at 4° C
   B. incubated at 37° C
   C. refrigerated in a deep freezer
   D. refrigerated for the initial three hours and then incubated at 37° C

12. A premature infant is delivered at 27 weeks of gestation and weighs 1,500 grams. How soon should the fundus examination be done by the ophthalmologist? 12.____

   A. Immediately
   B. 3-4 weeks after delivery
   C. At 34 weeks gestational age
   D. At 40 weeks gestational age

13. The most critical and constant finding in retinitis pigmentosa is 13.____

   A. dense bony spicule pigmentation in retinal periphery
   B. abnormal rhodopsin gene
   C. color blindness
   D. a significantly reduced electro-retinogram

14. Macular function tests include 14.____

   A. laser interferometry
   B. focal ERG
   C. electrocardiogram
   D. two point discrimination test

15. Fundus finding in a 40-year-old male shows bony spicule pigmentation in the retinal periphery, pale disc and attenuated retinal arterioles: 15.____

   A. retinitis pigmentosa
   B. diabetic retinopathy
   C. central serous retinopathy
   D. hypertensive retinopathy

16. Lattice degeneration is seen in 16.____

A. myopia
B. hypermetropia
C. retinitis pigmentosa
D. presbyopia

17. In diabetic retinopathy, ETDRS stands for 17.____

A. early treatment for diabetic retinopathy study
B. extended therapy for diabetic retinopathy and its study
C. early test for diabetic retinopathy and study
D. emergency treatment for diabetic retinopathy and its study

18. A young male of competitive nature comes to an ophthalmologist with sudden onset of blurring or decrease in vision in one eye and says it is painless. He improves spontaneously after three months. The likely cause is 18.____

A. macular hole
B. vitreous hemorrhage
C. central serous retinopathy
D. retinal detachment

19. Fundus examination should be done in a maturity onset diabetes mellitus patient ______ diagnosis. 19.____

A. at the time of
B. two years after
C. five years after
D. ten years after

20. Fluoroscein angiography is used to study the abnormality in all of the following EXCEPT the 20.____

A. retina
B. iris
C. lens
D. optic nerve head

21. Amsler's grid is useful in assessing 21.____

A. squint
B. macular function
C. depth of the anterior chamber
D. field of vision

22. Cherry red spot at the macula is seen in 22.____

A. CRAO
B. CRVO
C. myopia
D. ARMD

23. Cattle truck appearance on a fundoscopy is seen in 23.____

A. central retinal artery occlusion
B. diabetes mellitus
C. central serous retinopathy
D. syphilis

24. Angioid streaks are seen in 24.____

A. senile cataracts
B. open angle glaucoma
C. Eales' disease
D. pseudoxanthoma elasticum

25. Forster-Fuchs flecks are seen in 25.____

A. hypermetropia
B. degenerative myopia
C. gyrate atrophy of the retina
D. age-related macular degeneration

26. During fluorescein angiography, dye is injected into the 26.____

A. antecubital vein
B. carotid artery
C. saphenous vein
D. ophthalmic vein

27. Photoretinitis affects the 27.____

A. macula
B. optic disc
C. uvea
D. cornea

28. The development of ROP is highly correlated with 28.____

A. age of the mother
B. younger gestational age of child at birth
C. intrauterine growth retardation
D. immature retinal vasculature in zone III

29. Persistent hyperplastic primary vitreous is NOT associated with which one of the following? 29.____

A. Cataract
B. Peripheral retinal neovacularisation
C. Microphthalmos
D. Retinal detachment

30. The investigation of choice in young myopes with sudden appearance of black floaters in the eye is 30.____

A. retinoscopy
B. direct ophthalmoscopy
C. synoptophore examination
D. indirect ophthalmoscopy

31. Uhthoff's sign is seen in 31.____

A. diabetic retinopathy
B. multiple sclerosis
C. craniopharyngioma
D. diabetes insipidus

32. Toxic amblyopia is caused by which of the following? 32.____

A. Vitamin B-12
B. Ethambutol
C. Rifampicin
D. Pyrizinamide

33. Optic nerve axons emerge from 33.____

A. ganglion cells
B. rods and cones
C. amacrine cells
D. the outer nuclear layer

34. Leber's optic neuropathy has all of the following features EXCEPT 34.____

A. affected men do not pass the disease to their offspring; only women can
B. the visual loss is uniocular, sudden, painless, progressive and permanent

C. pupillary reflexes are affected early in the disease
D. typical visual field defects are centrocaecal

35. Papilledema is associated with all of the following changes EXCEPT 35.____

A. inflammation
B. vascular changes
C. edema of the optic nerve head and peripapillary area
D. forward bowing of the anterior part of lamina cribrosa

36. Double floor sign in a skull X-ray is found in 36.____

A. optic nerve glioma
B. meningioma
C. pituitary adenoma
D. carotid aneurysm

37. Suprasellar calcification is found in an X-ray of someone with 37.____

A. craniopharyngioma
B. meningioma
C. pituitary adenoma
D. third ventricle expansion

38. Anterior knee of Wilbrand is the 38.____

A. anterior extension of the superonasal chiasmal fibers crossing into the opposite optic tract
B. anterior extension of the inferonasal chiasmal fibers crossing into the opposite optic nerve
C. loop formed by papillary fibers
D. anterior extension of optic radiation

39. Blood is supplied to the tip of the calcarine cortex by the ______ artery. 39.____

A. middle cerebral
B. posterior cerebral
C. posterior cerebellar
D. anterior cerebellar

40. Significant loss of vision in a patient with hypertension can occur due to all of the following EXCEPT 40.____

A. occipital ischemia
B. anterior ischemic optic neuropathy
C. papilloedema
D. retinal hemorrhage

41. All of the following are characteristics of optic neuritis EXCEPT 41.____

A. decreased visual acuity
B. decreased pupillary reflex
C. abnormal electroretinogram
D. abnormal visual evoked response

42. A chalky white optic disc is present in all of the following EXCEPT 42.____

A. syphilis
B. Leber's hereditary optic neuropathy
C. post papilloedema
D. traumatic avulsion of optic disc

43. In a normal human eye, the visual field is least 43.____

A. nasally
B. superiorly
C. temporally
D. inferiorly

44. Ipsilateral optic atrophy with contralateral papilloedema is a feature of 44.____

A. Fisher syndrome
B. Foster Kennedy syndrome
C. Vogt-Koyonagi-Harada syndrome
D. benign intracranial hypertension

45. All of the following can cause optic neuritis EXCEPT 45.____

A. rifampicin
B. digitalis
C. chloroquine
D. ethambutol

46. In cortical blindness, 46.____

A. direct and consensual reflex is absent in both eyes
B. direct and consensual reflex is present in both eyes
C. direct reflex is present while consensual reflex is absent on affected side
D. direct reflex is absent while consensual reflex is present on affected side

47. The optic nerve is vulnerable to injury with surgery on which of the following sinuses? 47.____

A. Frontal
B. Ethmoid
C. Maxillary
D. Sphenoid

48. Cone density is greatest in which part of the retina? 48.____

A. Macula
B. Peripapillary region
C. Arcuate region
D. Peripheral retina

49. Protanopia is due to color blindness for 49.____

A. red
B. green
C. blue
D. yellow

50. Tests for color blindness include all of the following EXCEPT the 50.____

A. Ishihara test
B. Farnsworth Munsell 100 hue test
C. Edridge Green lantern test
D. Synoptophore examination

KEY (CORRECT ANSWERS)

1.	B	11.	A	21.	B	31.	B	41.	C
2.	D	12.	A	22.	A	32.	B	42.	D
3.	C	13.	D	23.	A	33.	A	43.	A
4.	B	14.	C	24.	D	34.	C	44.	B
5.	B	15.	A	25.	B	35.	A	45.	A
6.	B	16.	A	26.	A	36.	C	46.	B
7.	D	17.	A	27.	A	37.	A	47.	D
8.	B	18.	C	28.	B	38.	B	48.	A
9.	C	19.	A	29.	B	39.	A	49.	A
10.	D	20.	C	30.	D	40.	C	50.	D

EXAMINATION SECTION
TEST 1

DIRECTIONS: Each question or incomplete statement is followed by several suggested answers or completions. Select the one that BEST answers the question or completes the statement. *PRINT THE LETTER OF THE CORRECT ANSWER IN THE SPACE AT THE RIGHT.*

1. The degree of hypermetropia corrected by a patient's accommodative effort is called 1.____

   A. facultative B. absolute
   C. manifest D. latent

2. The hypermetropia corrected by the inherent tone of ciliary muscle is called 2.____

   A. facultative B. absolute
   C. manifest D. latent

3. Pathological hypermetropia may be due to 3.____

   A. deformational change in globe
   B. curvature change in the cornea
   C. absence of lens
   D. all of the above

4. In a hypermetropic person, on direct ophthalmoscopy, the image of observed fundus is 4.____

   A. equal to the size of part of the fundus observed
   B. smaller than the size of part of the fundus observed
   C. larger than the size of part of the fundus observed
   D. blurred

5. Which of the following statements is incorrect when retinoscopy is done using plane mirror? Movement of illuminated spot on fundus (seen in pupillary plane) is in the 5.____

   A. same direction as the immediate source of light in emmetropia
   B. same direction as the immediate source of light in hypermetropia
   C. opposite direction as the immediate source of light in myopia less than 1D
   D. opposite direction as the immediate source of light in myopia more than 1D

6. Which of the following statements is incorrect when retinoscopy is done using concave mirror? Movement of illuminated spot on fundus (seen in pupillary plane) is in the 6.____

   A. same direction as the immediate source of light in emmetropia
   B. same direction as the immediate source of light in hypermetropia
   C. opposite direction as the immediate source of light in myopia less than 1D
   D. opposite direction as the immediate source of light in myopia more than 1D

7. Distant direct ophthalmoscopy is done at 7.____

   A. 10 cm B. 25 cm C. 50 cm D. 1 m

8. In a hypermetrope, which of the following is incorrect? 8.____

   A. The eye is large
   B. Angle of anterior chamber is narrow

C. The cornea is small
D. Anterior chamber is shallow

9. Fundus finding in a hypermetrope include 9.____

A. shot silk appearance
B. optic neuritis like picture
C. small optic disc
D. all of the above

10. Ocular changes in myopia include all of the following EXCEPT 10.____

A. large eyeball
B. chorioretinal thinning
C. shallow anterior chamber
D. oval appearance of optic disc

11. Posterior segment changes of myopia include all of the following EXCEPT 11.____

A. myopic crescent in fundus
B. supertraction of retina on nasal side of optic disc
C. posterior staphyloma
D. choroidal thickening

12. Management of high myopia does NOT include 12.____

A. genetic counseling
B. contact lens
C. topical steroids
D. radial keratotomy

13. Uncorrected ametropia can cause all of the following EXCEPT 13.____

A. visual strain
B. squint
C. amblyopia
D. cataract

14. Diagnosis of astigmatism can be made by all of the following EXCEPT 14.____

A. placido disc
B. keratometry
C. videokeratography
D. direct ophthalmoscopy

15. The type of astigmatism in which two meridians are not horizontal and vertical though still at right angles to each other is called _______ astigmatism. 15.____

A. with the rule
B. against the rule
C. oblique
D. irregular

16. Clinical features of keratoconus include all of the following EXCEPT 16.____

A. Fleischer's ring
B. increased visibility of corneal nerves
C. irregular astigmatism
D. frequent perforations of the cornea

17. Which of the following has the greatest refractive power? 17.____

A. Anterior surface of the cornea
B. Posterior surface of the cornea
C. Anterior surface of the lens

D. Posterior surface of the lens

18. In myopia, which type of staphyloma is most common? 18.____

A. Equatorial
B. Posterior
C. Ciliary
D. Intercalary

19. One millimeter increase or decrease in axial length is equivalent to how many dioptres? 19.____

A. 1
B. 2
C. 3
D. 4

20. The eye of the newborn is 20.____

A. hypermetrope with regular astigmatism
B. hypermetrope
C. hypermetrope with irregular astigmatism
D. myopia

21. Diopteric power of the cornea is 21.____

A. +38 D
B. +40 D
C. +43 D
D. +48 D

22. Landolt's broken ring is used for testing 22.____

A. visual fields
B. visual acuity
C. angle of squint
D. for diagnosis of nystagmus

23. All of the following will seek early help for presbyopia symptoms EXCEPT a 23.____

A. short person
B. jeweller
C. hyperope
D. myope

24. The need for presbyopia glasses in a myope may be 24.____

A. delayed
B. earlier
C. unaffected
D. at the same time as in a hypermetrope

25. Presbyopia can be corrected by all EXCEPT 25.____

A. LASIK
B. glasses
C. contact lenses
D. convergence exercises

26. Physiological tone of ciliary muscle is 26.____

A. 1.0 D
B. 1.5 D
C. 2.0 D
D. 2.5 D

27. Causes of presbyopia include all of the following EXCEPT 27.____

A. the lens becoming harder and less moldable
B. weakness of the ciliary muscle
C. reduction in circumlental space
D. increase in curvature of the cornea

28. What is the power of the presbyopic spectacle to be used in a 45-year-old who has been emmetropic? 28.____

A. +1.5 D
B. +1.0 D
C. +2.0 D
D. +2.5 D

29. Treatment remedies for presbyopia do NOT include 29.____

A. glasses
B. contact lenses
C. LASIK
D. penetrating keratoplasty

30. Causes for early onset of presbyopia include all of the following EXCEPT 30.____

A. open angle glaucoma
B. associated hypermetropia
C. poor nutrition
D. squint

31. All of the following are true regarding aphakia EXCEPT 31.____

A. image size increases by about 30%
B. accommodation is partially preserved due to intact ciliary muscle
C. the field of vision is greatly reduced
D. there is spherical aberration called pincushion distortion

32. Contact lenses do NOT provide which of the following advantages when used in treatment of aphakia? 32.____

A. Less aniseikonia
B. Elimination of prismatic effect of aphakic glasses
C. Less incidence of ocular infections
D. Bigger and better field of vision

33. Which of the following statements is false? 33.____

A. Magnification of an image with use of a contact lens in an aphakic eye is 10-13%
B. Magnification of an image with use of a posterior chamber implant in an aphakic eye is 0.2%
C. Magnification of an image with use of aphakic glasses in an aphakic eye is 30%
D. With an intraocular lens, an additional advantage is that accommodation is retained

34. Factors affecting surgically induced astigmatism do NOT include 34.____

A. size and material of suture used
B. size of wound
C. age of patient
D. depth of suture

35. Causes of aniseikonia are 35.____

A. optical, i.e. difference in diopteric system of eyes
B. anatomical, i.e. displacement of retinal elements
C. central, i.e. asymmetrical simultaneous perception by brain
D. all of the above

KEY (CORRECT ANSWERS)

1. A
2. D
3. D
4. B
5. C

6. C
7. B
8. A
9. D
10. C

11. D
12. C
13. D
14. D
15. C

16. D
17. A
18. B
19. C
20. B

21. C
22. B
23. D
24. A
25. D

26. A
27. D
28. A
29. D
30. D

31. B
32. C
33. D
34. C
35. D

TEST 2

DIRECTIONS: Each question or incomplete statement is followed by several suggested answers or completions. Select the one that BEST answers the question or completes the statement. *PRINT THE LETTER OF THE CORRECT ANSWER IN THE SPACE AT THE RIGHT.*

1. Which of the following values is not needed for calculation of power of the intraocular lens? 1.____

   A. Axial length
   B. Keratometry
   C. Specific constant for each lens type
   D. Measure of amount of ocular movements

2. Low vision aids are not indicated in which of the following conditions? 2.____

   A. Age-related macular degeneration
   B. High myopia
   C. Retinitis pigmentosa
   D. Corneal opacity

3. The principles used in low vision aids are 3.____

   A. bringing the objects nearer
   B. magnification of retinal image
   C. increasing the size of the object to be viewed
   D. all of the above

4. Among these low vision aids, magnification of the retinal image is done in all of the following EXCEPT 4.____

   A. Fresnel lens
   B. Hastings triplet
   C. stenopaeic glasses
   D. biconvex lens (ex.+16D lens)

5. Of the following, which is NOT a non-optical low vision aid? 5.____

   A. Stand magnifier
   B. Special books with larger print
   C. Projection devices like closed-circuit TV with magnified image on the monitor
   D. Talking book

6. Which statement is NOT true of age-related macular degeneration? 6.____

   A. In confluent soft drusens, fluoroscein angiography should be done
   B. Dry ARMD is more dangerous than wet ARMD
   C. Photodynamic therapy should be done for subretinal neovascularization
   D. Transpupillary thermotherapy should be done for occult subretinal neovascular membrane

7. Which of the following correctly indicates pathological myopia? 7.____

   A. >-1D
   B. >-2D
   C. >-4D
   D. >-6D

8. Which statement is correct regarding macular diseases? 8.____

A. Flash ERG amplitude is decreased
B. EOG ratio is abnormal
C. Pattern ERG amplitude is decreased
D. None of the above

9. Retinal changes in myopia do not include 9.____

A. hole
B. paving stone degeneration
C. lattice degeneration
D. pseudoneuritic optic disc

10. Retinal pigment epithelial transplantation intravitreally is used for treatment of 10.____

A. retinitis pigmentosa
B. high myopia
C. ARMD
D. open angle glaucoma

11. Fluoroscein angiography is indicated in retinitis pigmentosa to detect 11.____

A. cystoid macular edema
B. leaks from arterioles
C. neovascularization of disc
D. neovascularization elsewhere

12. Which of the following is not a motor adaptation to squint? 12.____

A. Fusion
B. Head posture
C. Blind spot mechanism
D. Nystagmus

13. Which is not true of suppression? 13.____

A. Needs a large angle deviation
B. Needs a constant deviation
C. Occurs early in childhood
D. Occurs in monocular condition

14. Amblyopia may be due to 14.____

A. strabismus
B. anisometropia
C. form vision deprivation
D. all of the above

15. Which of the following is true of anomalous retinal correspondence? 15.____

A. Objective angle equals subjective angle
B. Objective angle is more than subjective angle
C. Occurs in intermittent squint
D. Occurs in late onset squint

16. Diagnosis of anomalous retinal correspondence can be done by all of the following EXCEPT 16.____

A. synoptophore
B. after-image test
C. Ishihara's color plate
D. Worth four dot test

17. Treatment of amblyopia does not include 17.____

A. retinal laser treatment
B. occlusion
C. inverse occlusion
D. carbidopa

18. In grades of binocular vision, grade 2 is 18.____

A. simultaneous macular perception
B. fusion
C. stereopsis
D. suppression

19. Hirschberg's test is used to detect 19.____

A. squint
B. field defect
C. glaucoma
D. optic atrophy

20. A large positive kappa angle simulates 20.____

A. esotropia
B. exotropia
C. hypertropia
D. hypotropia

21. All of the following are features of paralytic squint of adult onset EXCEPT 21.____

A. restricted eye movements
B. diplopia
C. change in head posture
D. amblyopia

22. The cover-uncover test is used to diagnose 22.____

A. heterotropia
B. heterophoria
C. childhood esotropia
D. infantile exotropia

23. Maddox wing is used to determine the amount of 23.____

A. heterotropia
B. heterophoria
C. hypertropia
D. hypotropia

24. Maddox rod is a series of fused 24.____

A. white cylindrical glasses
B. red cylindrical glasses
C. prisms of increasing strength
D. alternating spherical and cylindrical glasses

25. All of the following are used to detect diplopia EXCEPT 25.____

A. Hess chart
B. Lees screen
C. prism bar cover test
D. Maddox rod

26. The best treatment for amblyopia is 26.____

A. orthoptic exercise
B. occlusion
C. squint correction
D. carbidopa

27. Concomitant squint is different from paralytic squint in that 27.____

A. there is limitation of ocular movements
B. head tilting is frequent
C. the angle of squint is the same in all cardinal positions
D. diplopia is frequent

28. Double elevator palsy of the right eye is due to paresis of the 28.____

A. superior rectus of the right eye and inferior oblique muscle of the left eye
B. bilateral superior rectus
C. bilateral inferior oblique
D. superior rectus and inferior oblique muscle of the right eye

29. Childhood squint surgery is best done at 29.____

A. birth
B. 10 years
C. 15 years
D. 5 years

30. In paralytic squint, 30.____

A. primary deviation > secondary deviation
B. primary deviation < secondary deviation
C. primary deviation = secondary deviation
D. none of the above

31. Third nerve palsy, during early period, is associated with 31.____

A. uncrossed diplopia
B. crossed diplopia
C. amblyopia
D. none of the above

32. Which of the following is true about latent squint? 32.____

A. It is clinically called tropias
B. Detected by cover-uncover test
C. It is always convergent
D. It is always associated with decreased vision

33. Brown's syndrome simulates paresis of which of the following muscles? 33.____

A. Superior oblique
B. Inferior oblique
C. Inferior rectus
D. Superior rectus

34. Uncrossed diplopia is seen in 34.____

A. exotropia
B. exophoria
C. esotropia
D. esophoria

35. Third nerve palsy causes all of the following EXCEPT 35.____

A. ptosis
B. pupillary dilatation
C. medial deviation of the eyeball
D. loss of pupillary reflex

KEY (CORRECT ANSWERS)

1. D
2. D
3. D
4. C
5. A

6. B
7. D
8. C
9. D
10. A

11. A
12. D
13. D
14. D
15. B

16. C
17. A
18. B
19. A
20. B

21. D
22. B
23. B
24. B
25. C

26. B
27. C
28. D
29. D
30. B

31. B
32. B
33. B
34. C
35. C

TEST 3

DIRECTIONS: Each question or incomplete statement is followed by several suggested answers or completions. Select the one that BEST answers the question or completes the statement. *PRINT THE LETTER OF THE CORRECT ANSWER IN THE SPACE AT THE RIGHT.*

1. A 4-year-old child has a left convergent squint of six months duration. What is the appropriate management of this condition? 1.____

   A. Immediate surgical correction followed by amblyopia therapy
   B. Proper refractive correction, amblyopia therapy followed by surgical correction
   C. Prescribe spectacles and defer surgery until the child is age 5
   D. Botulinum toxin injection followed by occlusion therapy

2. Which of the following is NOT a clinical feature of right-sided VI nerve palsy? 2.____

   A. Medial convergent squint
   B. Face turn toward left
   C. Diplopia
   D. Inability to abduct right eye

3. Internuclear ophthalmoplegia is due to the lesion of the 3.____

   A. PPRF
   B. medial longitudinal fasciculus
   C. optic radiation
   D. lateral geniculate body

4. The most common complication of botulinum toxin injection is 4.____

   A. eyelid ptosis
   B. globe perforation
   C. retrobulbar hemorrhage
   D. vertical strabismus

5. To which of the following does Hering's law NOT apply? 5.____

   A. Version movements
   B. Inhibitional palsy
   C. Primary and secondary deviations
   D. Co-contraction of horizontal muscles in Duane syndrome

6. The first treatment for an accommodative esotropia is 6.____

   A. full refractive correction B. surgery
   C. amblyopia therapy D. orthoptic exercises

7. Overcorrection of myopia can cause 7.____

   A. accommodative spasm in the subject
   B. accommodative paralysis in the subject
   C. no effect on accommodation
   D. convergence insufficiency

8. Causes of cycloplegia include all of the following EXCEPT 8.____

   A. atropine
   B. diphtheria
   C. herpes zoster ophthalmicus
   D. myasthenia gravis

9. Which of the following drugs causes accommodative spasm? 9.____

   A. Echothiophate diisopropyl-fluorophosphate
   B. Atropine
   C. Tropicamide
   D. Diamox

10. Which of the following does NOT have an associated accommodative insufficiency? 10.____

    A. Presbyopia
    B. Debilitating disease
    C. Use of miotics
    D. Anemia

11. Which of these formulas gives the amount of accommodation appropriate for age (in years)? 11.____

    A. 4x4- age / 4
    B. 4-age/4
    C. 4 x 4 - age
    D. 4-age

12. The measuring unit of convergence is 12.____

    A. meter
    B. degree
    C. meter angle
    D. prism dioptre

13. The ratio of AC:A is 13.____

    A. 2:3
    B. 3:2
    C. 4:1
    D. 5:1

14. Treatment of refractive accommodative esotropia is 14.____

    A. orthoptic exercises
    B. surgery
    C. full spectacle correction
    D. all of the above

15. The power f accommodation in a child with a punctum proximum situated at 7 cm is 15.____

    A. +14D
    B. +10D
    C. +12D
    D. +7D

16. LASIK can correct all of the following EXCEPT 16.____

    A. myopia
    B. hypermetropia
    C. cataract
    D. astigmatism

17. Myopia is corrected by 17.____

    A. radial keratotomy
    B. LASIK
    C. removal of clear lens
    D. all of the above

18. Photorefractive keratectomy is not indicated in 18.____

    A. myopia < 6D
    B. hypermetropia < 2D
    C. astigmatism < 0.5D
    D. keratoconus

19. Which of the following tests is not useful in subjective verification of refraction? 19.____

A. Acceptance
B. Duochrome
C. Astigmatic fan
D. Synoptophore examination

20. For retinoscopy, 20._____

A. accommodation should be partially relaxed
B. accommodation should be completely relaxed
C. accommodation should not be relaxed
D. the person should be fully accommodating

21. The trial case does NOT contain 21._____

A. a pair of plus spheres ranging from +0.12D to +20.0D
B. a pair of minus spheres ranging from -0.12D to -20.0D
C. fluoroscein strips
D. a pair of plus and minus cylinders ranging from 0.12D to 8.0D

22. The longest time for onset of cycloplegia is taken by 22._____

A. atropine
B. homatropine
C. cyclopentolate
D. tropicamide

23. Dynamic retinoscopy is also called 23._____

A. dry retinoscopy
B. static retinoscopy
C. retinoscopy with cycloplegia
D. none of the above

24. Most automated refractors utilize 24._____

A. UV light
B. normal light
C. infrared light source
D. red light

25. All of the following methods are used to check astigmatism EXCEPT 25._____

A. astigmatic fan
B. cross cylinders of Jackson
C. keratometry
D. indirect ophthalmoscopy

26. Tests for malingering include all of the following EXCEPT 26._____

A. menace reflex
B. opticokinetic nystagmus
C. objective fixation test with use of prisms
D. testing visual acuity with Snellen's chart

27. Which type of LASIK is used to correct high order aberrations? 27._____

A. Presbyopic
B. Astigmatic
C. Myopic
D. Customized

28. Which statement is correct for hyperopic LASIK? 28._____

A. Peripheral laser pulses are needed to flatten peripheral cornea
B. Small diameter flap is needed
C. Central cornea is flattened
D. Hyperopia up to +10D can be corrected

29. Which is NOT an advantage of phakic IOL? 29.____

A. Reversibility
B. Immediate correction
C. Stability
D. Cataract formation

30. In children under 2 years of age, at the time of surgery for congenital cataract, the power of IOL to be inserted is reduced from that estimated by A scan by 30.____

A. 20%
B. 10%
C. 5%
D. not to be reduced

31. Advantages of LASEK include all of the following EXCEPT 31.____

A. more post-operative pain
B. less post-operative haze
C. suitable in patients with narrow palpebral aperture
D. useful in patients with thin cornea

32. The refractive index of the cornea is 32.____

A. 1.33 B. 1.37 C. 1.42 D. 1.44

33. The power of reduced eye is normally 33.____

A. 20D B. 38D C. 18D D. 60D

34. In a Goldman single-mirror gonioscope, the mirror is placed at an angle to the flat surface measuring 34.____

A. 64 B. 50 C. 23 D. 15

35. In a Goldman three-mirror contact lens, the 73 inclined mirror is used to examine 35.____

A. posterior pole of the eye
B. macula to 30°
C. 30° to equator
D. ora serrata

36. A focimeter is used for 36.____

A. calculating the anterior focal point of the eye
B. calculating the posterior focal point of the eye
C. calculating the spherical and cylindrical power of the glasses
D. measuring the power of the anterior corneal surface

37. All of the following are contraindications to the use of contact lenses EXCEPT 37.____

A. keratitis
B. giant papillary conjunctivitis
C. squint
D. dusty environmental conditions

38. Distant direct ophthalmoscopy is done at 38.____

A. 10 cm B. 25 cm C. 50 cm D. 1 m

39. Optical indications of contact lenses include all of the following EXCEPT 39.____

A. myopia
B. hyperopia
C. unsightly corneas or eyeball
D. albinism

40. Complications of contact lenses include all of the following EXCEPT 40.____

A. lens splitting
B. tight lens syndrome
C. lens spoilage with deposits
D. all of the above

KEY (CORRECT ANSWERS)

1. B	11. A	21. C	31. A
2. B	12. C	22. A	32. B
3. B	13. C	23. A	33. D
4. A	14. C	24. C	34. A
5. D	15. A	25. D	35. B
6. A	16. C	26. D	36. C
7. A	17. D	27. D	37. C
8. D	18. D	28. A	38. B
9. A	19. D	29. D	39. C
10. C	20. B	30. A	40. D

EXAMINATION SECTION
TEST 1

DIRECTIONS: Each question or incomplete statement is followed by several suggested answers or completions. Select the one that BEST answers the question or completes the statement. *PRINT THE LETTER OF THE CORRECT ANSWER IN THE SPACE AT THE RIGHT.*

1. Which of the following factors contributes MOST to infant mortality? 1____

   A. Motor vehicle accidents
   B. Congenital cardiac malformation
   C. Prematurity
   D. Acute renal failure
   E. Pneumonia

2. All of the following statements are true regarding tuberculosis in the United States EXCEPT: 2____

   A. Mortality and morbidity rates increase with age
   B. Mortality rates are higher for males than females
   C. The incidence is much higher among the poor than the rich
   D. In low incidence areas, such as the United States, most tuberculosis is exogenous
   E. In 2015, the reported incidence of clinical disease in the United States was 3.0/100,000 population

3. Tubercle bacilli CANNOT be destroyed by 3____

   A. heat
   B. cold
   C. ultraviolet light
   D. phenol
   E. tricresol solution

4. The MOST frequent reservoirs for tuberculosis disease are 4____

   A. badgers
   B. mosquitoes
   C. humans
   D. cats
   E. deer

5. The LEADING cause of death for people younger than age 65 in the United States is 5____

   A. heart disease
   B. cerebrovascular disease
   C. chronic obstructive pulmonary disease
   D. diabetes mellitus
   E. chronic liver disease

6. Cooling towers and air conditioning units serve as breeding grounds for 6____

   A. staphylococcus aureus
   B. klebsiella pneumoniae
   C. streptococcus pneumoniae
   D. L. pneumophilia
   E. histoplasma capsulatum

7. Diseases transmitted by mosquitoes, mites, and ticks can be prevented by all of the following precautions EXCEPT 7_____

A. protective clothing
B. mask and gloves
C. insect repellents
D. door and window screens
E. more than one but not all of the above

8. The PRINCIPAL area of study in injury control is 8_____

A. epidemiology
B. prevention
C. treatment
D. rehabilitation
E. all of the above

9. Benzene is MOST likely to be associated with ______ cancer. 9_____

A. blood
B. kidney
C. liver
D. brain
E. bone

10. A ______ test is used when the patient's wishes can be inferred from his or her known religious, ethical, and/or lifestyle beliefs. 10_____

A. subjective
B. relative
C. limited objective
D. pure objective
E. none of the above

11. It is NOT true that standard deviation 11_____

A. is the positive square root of variance
B. is the most useful measure of dispersion
C. standardizes extreme values
D. decreases when the sample size increases
E. of a small size in a sample causes the sample mean to be close to each individual value

12. The difference between the highest and lowest values in a series is called the 12_____

A. range
B. variance
C. standard deviation
D. coefficient of variation
E. none of the above

13. The ratio of the standard deviation of a series to the arithmetic mean of the series is known as the 13_____

A. coefficient of variation
B. range
C. variance
D. frequency
E. prevalence

14. In a disease which is usually of acute onset, lasts a couple of weeks, and has a case fatality rate of 75 to 85%, the 14_____

A. prevalence is always higher than that of annual incidence
B. incidence is always higher than the prevalence
C. prevalence and annual incidence are always equal
D. mortality rate will be consistently high in all countries where the disease occurs
E. none of the above

15. A random sample of 20,000 men is screened for a history of excessive sugar consumption and the presence of diabetes. 15_____
This is called a ______ study.

A. prospective
B. historical
C. cross-sectional population
D. retrospective-prospective
E. case control retrospective

16. Five hundred young adults who are known cocaine users are assembled together with a control group. Recognizable psychotics are excluded, and the remainder are followed for 3 years to see whether any psychoses develop in them. 16_____
This is a ______ study.

A. retrospective
B. case control retrospective
C. cross-sectional population
D. cohort
E. none of the above

17. The FIRST and most important thing for the epidemiologist to do during the investigation of a patient with a communicable disease is to investigate 17_____

A. the first source of infection
B. the mode of transmission
C. how many people have been infected
D. the accuracy of the diagnosis
E. preventive control of the disease

18. The single MOST important measure for the prevention of typhoid fever in a community is 18_____

A. a ceftriaxon prophylaxis for all persons who are exposed to the disease
B. washing hands
C. immunization of the high risk population
D. hospitalization and treatment of all known carriers
E. water purification

19. Diseases more likely to occur in women than in men include all of the following EXCEPT 19_____

A. Raynaud's disease
B. sarcoidosis
C. gout
D. systemic lupus erythematosus
E. secondary hypothyroidism

20. Over the past 50 years, which of the following chronic conditions has experienced the greatest decline in mortality rate? 20_____

A. Heart disease
B. Stroke
C. Cancer
D. Pneumonia
E. Influenza

21. The population having the HIGHEST frequency of thalassemia is the 21____

A. Jews
B. Italians
C. Chinese
D. Japanese
E. Americans

22. Over the past ten years, the majority of individuals who were initially diagnosed with diabetes mellitus were in what age group? 22____

A. 18-29
B. 30-39
C. 50-59
D. 70-79
E. 80-89

23. Of the following, the disease LARGELY confined to people born in temperate climate zones and manifested in early adult life is 23____

A. diabetes
B. multiple sclerosis
C. thalassemia
D. hypertension
E. prostate cancer

24. Hepatitis A has the highest incidence rate in individuals in which age group? 24____

A. 0-9
B. 10-19
C. 20-29
D. 30-39
E. 50-59

25. Recurrent episodes of low grade fever and arthralgia FREQUENTLY affect workers in 25____

A. slaughter houses
B. cotton mills
C. coal mines
D. hospital laboratories
E. none of the above

KEY (CORRECT ANSWERS)

1. C
2. D
3. B
4. C
5. A
6. D
7. B
8. E
9. A
10. C
11. C
12. A
13. A
14. B
15. C
16. D
17. D
18. E
19. C
20. B
21. B
22. C
23. B
24. C
25. A

TEST 2

DIRECTIONS: Each question or incomplete statement is followed by several suggested answers or completions. Select the one that BEST answers the question or completes the statement. *PRINT THE LETTER OF THE CORRECT ANSWER IN THE SPACE AT THE RIGHT.*

1. Risk factors for malignancies of the liver and intra-hepatic biliary tract may include all of the following EXCEPT 1____

   A. alpha-1 antitrypsin deficiency
   B. aflatoxin
   C. gentamicin
   D. alcohol
   E. steroids

2. The parasite associated with an increased risk for developing carcinoma of the biliary tree is 2____

   A. ascaris lumbricoides
   B. balantidium coli
   C. cryptoporidium
   D. colonorchis sinensis
   E. enterobias vermicular is

3. Of the following, the immunization that should NOT be given to an individual who has received immune globulin within the previous 3 months is 3____

   A. IPV
   B. DTP
   C. MMR
   D. HBIG
   E. none of the above

4. Which of the following is the LEADING cause of maternal death among pregnancies with abortive outcomes? 4____

   A. Rubella
   B. Ectopic pregnancy
   C. Teratoma
   D. Defective germ cell
   E. Herpes simplex II

5. All of the following are leading causes of maternal mortality in the United States EXCEPT 5____

   A. anesthesia complication
   B. embolism
   C. hypertensive disease of pregnancy
   D. hemorrhage
   E. maternal age between 20 and 30

6. _______ is NOT a reportable disease. 6____

   A. Pulmonary tuberculosis
   B. Mumps
   C. Measles
   D. Choriomeningitis
   E. Meningococcal sepsis

7. The scientific field dealing with the collection, classification, description, analysis, interpretation, and presentation of data is called 7____

   A. distributions
   B. statistics
   C. standard deviation
   D. median
   E. cohort study

8. What type of treatment regimen should be administered to an infant born to a mother with active gonorrhea? 8____

A. Single IM dose of ceftriaxone
B. Single oral dose of azithromycin
C. Dual therapy of ceftriaxone and azithromycin
D. Dual therapy of ceftriaxone and spectinomycin
E. None of the above

9. A precaution necessary for children in day care who have pneumococcal disease is ______ isolation. 9____

A. strict
B. contact
C. enteric
D. respiratory
E. none of the above

10. Children who have ever had a life-threatening allergic reaction to ________ should not get the polio vaccine. 10____

A. gluten
B. peanuts
C. eggs
D. antibiotics
E. pollen

11. Stillbirths or perinatal death is a result of ______ % of pregnancies in women with untreated early syphilis. 11____

A. 5
B. 10
C. 25
D. 40
E. 80

12. Strongyloidiasis is endemic in the tropics and subtropics, including the southern and southwestern United States. The single MOST important control measure is 12____

A. purification of water
B. food cooked at a higher temperature
C. sanitary disposal measure for human waste
D. mass vaccination of exposed population
E. detection and treatment of all infected persons

13. In a large population, the mode of transmission MOST difficult to prevent is ______ spread. 13____

A. vector
B. person to person
C. airborne
D. droplet
E. none of the above

14. Of the following, the factor contributing the MOST to infant mortality is 14____

A. seizures
B. prematurity
C. hypothyroidism
D. congenital heart disease
E. birth trauma

15. Point prevalence studies tend to have an over-representation of 15____

A. chronic cases
B. fatal cases
C. short-term cases
D. healthy persons
E. all of the above

16. The PRIMARY function of the federal government in the Medicaid program is to 16____

A. set standards
B. provide services in their own institutions *only*
C. investigate *only* services rendered
D. pay for services
E. pay for nursing care *only*

Questions 17-21.

DIRECTIONS: In Questions 17 through 21, match the numbered description with the appropriate lettered term listed in Column I. Place the letter of the correct answer in the space at the right.

<u>COLUMN I</u>

A. Sensitivity
B. Specificity
C. Screening
D. Median
E. Mode

17. The MOST commonly occurring value in a series of values 17____

18. The initial examination of an individual whose disease is not yet under medical care 18____

19. May be calculated in an ongoing longevity study 19____

20. The ability of a screening test to identify correctly those individuals who truly have the disease 20____

21. The ability of a test to identify correctly those individuals who truly do not have the disease 21____

Questions 22-25.

DIRECTIONS: In Questions 22 through 25, match the numbered definition with the appropriate lettered term listed in Column I. Place the letter of the correct answer in the space at the right.

<u>COLUMN I</u>

A. Efficiency
B. Validity
C. Reliability
D. Bias
E. Causality

22. The extent to which a test provides the same result on the same subject on two or more occasions 22____

23. The extent to which the results of a test agree with the results of another test that is accepted as more accurate or closer to the truth 23____

24. A systematic error that is unintentionally made 24____

25. Denotes direct effect 25____

KEY (CORRECT ANSWERS)

1. C
2. D
3. C
4. B
5. E

6. D
7. B
8. C
9. E
10. D

11. D
12. C
13. C
14. B
15. C

16. D
17. E
18. C
19. D
20. A

21. B
22. C
23. B
24. D
25. E

EXAMINATION SECTION
TEST 1

DIRECTIONS: Each question or incomplete statement is followed by several suggested answers or completions. Select the one that BEST answers the question or completes the statement. *PRINT THE LETTER OF THE CORRECT ANSWER IN THE SPACE AT THE RIGHT.*

Questions 1-4.

DIRECTIONS: Questions 1 through 4 are to be answered on the basis of the following information.

In a day care center of 30 children (20 females and 10 males), 7 boys develop hepatitis A over a 3-week period. During the next 8 weeks, an additional 2 boys and 5 girls develop the infection.

1. The attack rate of hepatitis A in this day care center is ______%. 1.____

   A. 20 B. 30 C. 40 D. 46.6 E. 54.5

2. The secondary attack rate of hepatitis A in this day care center is MOST NEARLY ______%. 2.____

   A. 20 B. 15 C. 23 D. 27 E. 10

3. The attack rate of hepatitis A for boys in this school is MOST NEARLY ______%. 3.____

   A. 16 B. 40 C. 50 D. 60 E. 64

4. The attack rate of hepatitis A for girls is MOST NEARLY ______%. 4.____

   A. 21 B. 24 C. 25 D. 27 E. 30

5. The epidemic curve suggests a common source outbreak with 5.____

   A. continuing common source outbreak
   B. fecal-oral transmission
   C. secondary airborne transmission
   D. secondary person-to-person transmission
   E. none of the above

6. The ______ rate is determined by the number of deaths caused by a specific disease divided by the number of cases of the disease. 6.____

   A. mortality
   B. case fatality
   C. attack
   D. cause specific death
   E. none of the above

7. Rate is the expression of the probability of occurrence of a particular event in a defined population during a specified period of time. 7.____
   The rate calculated for various segments of the population is known as the ______ rate.

   A. specific
   B. crude
   C. adjusted
   D. variable
   E. none of the above

8. The sources of disease surveillance data include all of the following EXCEPT 8.___

A. individual case reports
B. emergency room visit records
C. hospital discharge summaries
D. death certificates
E. none of the above

9. All of the following are true about tularemia EXCEPT that it is 9.___

A. a zoonotic disease
B. more common during the summer months in the western states
C. more common in winter months in the eastern states
D. primarily transmitted by the bite of a spider
E. none of the above

10. Which of the following is NOT among the basic steps in an investigation of an epidemic? 10.___

A. Verification of diagnosis
B. Establishing the existence of an epidemic
C. Characterization of the distribution of cases
D. Formulating a conclusion
E. All of the above

11. The LAST step in conducting an epidemic investigation is to 11.___

A. develop an hypothesis
B. test the hypothesis
C. formulate a conclusion
D. institute control measures
E. establish the diagnosis of an epidemic

12. The patients who are infected with an agent but never develop clinical symptoms of the disease are known as ______ carriers. 12.___

A. incubatory
B. subclinical
C. chronic
D. convalescent
E. clinical

13. All of the following are uses of epidemiology EXCEPT to 13.___

A. identify factors that cause disease
B. explain how and why diseases and epidemics occur
C. establish a clinical diagnosis of disease
D. determine a patient's prognosis
E. evaluate the effectiveness of health programs

14. The biological traits that determine the occurrence of a disease include all of the following EXCEPT 14.___

A. genetic characteristics
B. diet
C. race
D. ethnic origin
E. sex

15. The general factors of resistance in a human host include all of the following EXCEPT 15.____

A. the immune system
B. intact skin
C. diarrhea
D. normal bacterial flora
E. gastric juices

16. All of the following are examples of direct contact transmission EXCEPT 16.____

A. syphilis
B. herpes
C. hepatitis B
D. sporotrichosis
E. none of the above

17. The basic aims and specific goals of medical studies and clinical research do NOT include 17.____

A. assessing health status or clinical characteristics
B. eliminating all carriers of diseases
C. determining and assessing treatment outcomes
D. identifying and assessing risk factors
E. all of the above

18. Incidence and prevalence studies usually concern all of the following EXCEPT 18.____

A. the occurrence of disease
B. a comparison of outcomes between different treatments
C. adverse side effects of drugs
D. the death rate for a certain disease
E. none of the above

19. A case series report can address almost any clinical issue but it is MOST commonly used to describe 19.____

A. clinical characteristics of a disease
B. screening test results
C. treatment outcomes
D. an unexpected result or event
E. none of the above

20. A comparison of chemotherapy to chemotherapy plus radiation for laryngeal carcinoma would be an appropriate topic for a(n) 20.____

A. cohort study
B. case control study
C. clinical trial
D. case series report
E. incidence and prevalence study

21. The sum of all values in a series divided by the actual number of values in the series is known as the 21.____

A. mode
B. median
C. geometric mean
D. arithmetic mean
E. none of the above

22. The MOST commonly occurring value in a series of values is the 22.____

A. mode
B. median
C. geometric mean
D. arithmetic mean
E. none of the above

23. The ratio of the standard deviation of a series to the arithmetic mean of the series is known as the 23.____

A. range
B. variance
C. coefficient of variation
D. standard deviation
E. epidemic curve

24. The sum of squared deviations from the mean divided by the number of values in the series minus 1 is called the 24.____

A. range
B. variance
C. standard deviation
D. coefficient of variation
E. frequency polygon

25. The ______ is a tool for comparing categories of mutually exclusive discrete data. 25.____

A. pie chart
B. Venn diagram
C. bar diagram
D. histogram
E. frequency polygon

KEY (CORRECT ANSWERS)

1. D
2. C
3. E
4. C
5. D
6. B
7. A
8. E
9. D
10. E
11 D
12. B
13. D
14. B
15. A
16. E
17. B
18. B
19. A
20. C
21 D
22. A
23. C
24. B
25. C

TEST 2

DIRECTIONS: Each question or incomplete statement is followed by several suggested answers or completions. Select the one that BEST answers the question or completes the statement. *PRINT THE LETTER OF THE CORRECT ANSWER IN THE SPACE AT THE RIGHT.*

1. A ______ is a special form of the bar diagram used to represent categories of continuous and ordered data. 1.____

   A. pie chart
   B. histogram
   C. Venn diagram
   D. cumulative frequency graph
   E. frequency polygon

2. A medical student performs venipuncture on 1,000 randomly selected patients and is successful on the first attempt 700 times. 2.____
   What is the probability that her next venipuncture will be successful on the first attempt?

   A. 7% B. 14% C. 50% D. 70% E. 80%

3. All of the following are true regarding the standard error of the mean of a sample EXCEPT that it 3.____

   A. is an estimate of the standard deviation of the population
   B. is based on a normal distribution
   C. increases as the sample size increases
   D. is used to determine confidence limits
   E. none of the above

4. All of the following are characteristics of a confidence interval EXCEPT that it 4.____

   A. is based on a critical ratio when the sample is large
   B. gives an indication of the likely magnitude of the true value
   C. gives an indication of the certainty of the point estimate
   D. becomes narrower as the sample size increases
   E. none of the above

5. Nonparametric tests can be used to compare two populations with which of the following conditions? 5.____

   A. Each population is unimodal
   B. Both populations have equal numbers
   C. Each population is independent
   D. Each population is distributed normally
   E. All of the above

6. All of the following vaccines are grown in embryonated chicken eggs EXCEPT 6.____

   A. yellow fever B. measles C. mumps
   D. rubella E. influenza

7. Which of the following vaccines should NOT be given to individuals who live in households with an immuno-compromised host? 7.____

A. Yellow fever
B. Hepatitis B
C. Oral polio
D. Influenza
E. Diphtheriae

8. A solution of antibodies derived from the serum of animals immunized with a specific antigen is a(n) 8.____

A. immunoglobulin
B. antitoxin
C. toxoid
D. vaccine
E. none of the above

9. All of the following may be significant sequale of measles infection EXCEPT 9.____

A. pneumonia
B. encephalitis
C. congenital birth defects
D. mental retardation
E. death

10. All of the following statements about vaccination during pregnancy are true EXCEPT: 10.____

A. Live attenuated viral vaccines should not be given to pregnant women
B. Pregnant women at substantial risk of exposure may receive a live viral vaccine
C. There is evidence that inactivated vaccines also pose risks to the fetus
D. There is no evidence that immunoglobulins pose any risk to the fetus
E. None of the above

11. None of the following conditions are reasons for delaying or discontinuing routine immunizations EXCEPT 11.____

A. soreness, redness or swelling at the injection site in reaction to previous immunization
B. a temperature of more than 105F in reaction to previous DTP vaccine
C. mild diarrheal illness in an otherwise well child
D. current antimicrobial therapy
E. breastfeeding

12. Children and infants with any of the following disorders should not receive pertussis vaccine EXCEPT those with 12.____

A. uncontrolled epilepsy
B. infantile spasms
C. progressive encephalopathy
D. developmental delay
E. none of the above

13. Which of the following groups of patients should NOT receive pneumococcal polysaccharide vaccine? 13.____

A. Elderly, age 65 or older
B. Immunocompromised
C. Children age 2 years or older with anatomic or functional asplenia

D. Children age 2 years or older with nephrotic syndrome or CSF leaks
E. Children under 2 years of age

14. All of the following are significant complications of sexually transmitted diseases in women EXCEPT 14.____

A. pelvic inflammatory disease
B. infertility
C. teratogenicity
D. cancer
E. ectopic pregnancy

15. For primary prevention and maximal safety, a person should 15.____

A. engage in a mutually monogamous relationship
B. limit the number of sexual partners
C. inspect and question new partners
D. avoid sexual practices involving anal or fecal contact
E. all of the above

16. All of the following are complications caused by untreated syphilis infection EXCEPT 16.____

A. obesity
B. blindness
C. psychosis
D. cardiovascular disease
E. none of the above

17. All of the following statements are true regarding syphilis EXCEPT: 17.____

A. The organism cannot enter through intact skin
B. Everyone is susceptible
C. There is no natural or acquired immunity
D. No vaccine is available
E. Reinfection is rare

18. Which of the following sexually transmitted diseases rank as the number one reported communicable disease in the United States? 18.____

A. Syphilis
B. Gonorrhea
C. AIDS
D. Chlamydia
E. Hepatitis B

19. Which of the following is believed to be the MOST common sexually transmitted bacterial pathogen in the United States? 19.____

A. Treponema pallidum
B. Chlamydia trachomatis
C. Nisseriae gonorrhea
D. E. coli
E. Herpes zoster

20. All of the following are documented modes of transmission for human immunodeficiency virus EXCEPT ______ transmission. 20.____

A. sexual
B. percutaneous exposure
C. airborne
D. mother to child
E. none of the above

21. In order to prevent HIV infection, which of the following groups should NOT donate blood? 21.____

A. Any man who has had sexual contact with another man since 1977
B. Present or past IV drug abusers
C. Individuals from Central Africa and Haiti
D. Sexual partners of any of the above groups
E. All of the above

22. Chlamydia trachomatis, the causative agent of chlamydia infection, has all of the following characteristics EXCEPT it 22.____

A. grows only intracellularly
B. contains both DNA and RNA
C. is a protozoa
D. divides by binary fission
E. has cell walls similar to gram-negative bacteriae

23. All of the following are true regarding the resultant effects of chlamydia trachomatis EXCEPT: 23.____

A. Approximately 50% cases of non-gonococcal urethritis in men
B. 99% of cases of pelvic inflammatory disease
C. Mucopurulent cervicitis
D. Inclusion conjunctivitis in infants born to infected mothers
E. Acute epididymitis in men

24. All of the following statements are true regarding hepatitis A infection EXCEPT: 24.____

A. Approximately 70% of Americans are infected by the age of 20
B. Incidence appears to be declining
C. Infection is related to age and socioeconomic status
D. The incubation period is 15-50 days with an average of 28-30 days
E. Young children are more likely to have subclinical infections

25. The transmission of hepatitis A virus is facilitated by all of the following EXCEPT 25.____

A. poor personal hygiene
B. poor sanitation
C. drinking out of the same cup
D. eating uncooked or raw food
E. eating food contaminated by human hands after cooking

KEY (CORRECT ANSWERS)

1. B
2. D
3. C
4. E
5. E

6. D
7. C
8. B
9. C
10. C

11. B
12. D
13. E
14. C
15. E

16. A
17. E
18. B
19. B
20. C

21. E
22. C
23. B
24. A
25. C

EXAMINATION SECTION
TEST 1

DIRECTIONS: Each question or incomplete statement is followed by several suggested answers or completions. Select the one that BEST answers the question or completes the statement. *PRINT THE LETTER OF THE CORRECT ANSWER IN THE SPACE AT THE RIGHT.*

1. All of the following are characteristics of carbohydrates EXCEPT 1.____
   A. energy to the central nervous system
   B. necessary for the complete oxidation of fats
   C. they insulate and pad body organs
   D. grains, fruits, vegetables, milk, and sugar are common dietary sources

2. The MOST concentrated source of energy in food is in 2.____
   A. proteins B. carbohydrates
   C. vitamins D. lipids

3. Which of the following conditions may be caused by protein deficiencies? 3.____
   A. Kwashiorkor B. Marasmus
   C. Hypoproteinemia D. All of the above

4. All of the following are at risk for developing protein deficiencies EXCEPT 4.____
   A. strict vegetarians
   B. elderly persons on fixed incomes
   C. high-income families
   D. chronically ill

5. All of the following are fat soluble vitamins EXCEPT vitamin 5.____
   A. B_{12} B. D C. A D. K

6. A deficiency of vitamin ______ can cause night blindness. 6.____
   A. B_6 B. A C. C D. E

7. All of the following are common manifestations of vitamin D deficiency EXCEPT 7.____
   A. enlarged joints B. pernicious anemia
   C. delayed dentition D. rickets

8. All of the following are common functions of vitamin C EXCEPT 8.____
   A. synthesis of collagen
   B. facilitation of iron absorption
   C. maturation of red blood cells
   D. formation of intercellular cement

9. Of the following sources, what would you recommend a patient eat to get vitamin B_{12}? 9.____
   A. Milk B. Vegetables
   C. Citrus fruits D. Animal foods

10. The PREFERRED method of nutritional support for a malnourished patient with an intact gastrointestinal system is 10.____

    A. oral feeding
    B. tube feeding
    C. total parenteral nutrition
    D. peripheral vein parenteral nutrition

11. Bile is necessary for the absorption of 11.____

    A. thiamine (B_1)
    B. vitamin E
    C. riboflavin (B_2)
    D. vitamin C

12. A strict vegetarian diet often leads to a deficiency in vitamin 12.____

    A. C
    B. D
    C. E
    D. B_{12}

13. Which of the following is the BEST initial diet for a post-operative patient with vomiting and diarrhea? 13.____

    A. Low residue
    B. High fiber
    C. Clear liquid
    D. Gluten-free

14. The purpose of a low residue diet is to 14.____

    A. reduce the amount of indigestible fiber in the intestinal tract
    B. provide bulk in the stool
    C. eliminate lactose from the diet
    D. eliminate chemically irritating food from the diet to allow healing of gastric mucosa

15. The purpose of a renal diet is to control the intake of 15.____

    A. proteins
    B. fluids
    C. sodium and potassium
    D. all of the above

16. Which of the following minerals is the MAJOR constituent of hemoglobin? 16.____

    A. Calcium
    B. Iron
    C. Iodine
    D. Sodium

17. The causes of vitamin deficiency may include 17.____

    A. low intake
    B. failure of absorption
    C. increased demand or requirements
    D. all of the above

18. The clinical manifestations of calcium deficiency include all of the following EXCEPT 18.____

    A. tooth decay
    B. hoarseness and thick tongue
    C. nervousness and palpitations
    D. brittle fingernails and arm and leg numbness

19. All of the following are clinical manifestations of potassium deficiency EXCEPT 19.____

    A. muscle weakness
    B. cardiac arrest
    C. increased muscle tone
    D. mental confusion

20. The clinical manifestations of iodine deficiency may include 20.____

A. hypothyroidism
B. tachycardia
C. fever and profuse sweating
D. all of the above

21. Clinical manifestations of zinc deficiency include all of the following EXCEPT 21.____

A. poor wound healing
B. hypogonadism
C. hirsutism
D. loss of taste

22. Clinical indication of total parenteral nutrition (TPN) includes 22.____

A. chronic vomiting
B. stroke
C. chemotherapy or radiotherapy
D. all of the above

23. While feeding a patient with diarrhea, which of the following corrective measures should be taken? 23.____

A. Heat the formula to 100° C
B. Insert the feeding tube gently
C. Administer the formula slowly
D. All of the above

24. Which of the following data would support a nursing diagnosis of dehydration related to diarrhea? 24.____

A. Difficulty in breathing
B. Blood-stained urine
C. Urine output of 10 ml per hour
D. All of the above

25. A nurse observes a high hematocrit in a patient with vomiting and diarrhea. The MOST likely diagnosis is 25.____

A. leukopenia
B. volume depletion
C. bacterial infection
D. hypertension

26. In a patient with congestive heart failure, the nurse should advise 26.____

A. increasing caloric intake to gain weight
B. a single large meal daily
C. a sodium restricted diet
D. a high fat diet

27. A 4-month-old infant is admitted to the hospital with a diagnosis of rotavirus gastroenteritis with 10% dehydration. 27.____
The BEST method to observe the level of dehydration each shift is to assess his

A. capillary refill time
B. heart rate
C. weight
D. urine output

Questions 28-31.

DIRECTIONS: Questions 28 through 31 are to be answered on the basis of the following information.

An infant is admitted to the hospital with a diagnosis of failure to thrive.

28. The criteria used for this diagnosis includes all of the following EXCEPT 28.____

A. absence of organic disease
B. weight below 25th percentile with no subsequent weight gain when nurtured
C. developmental lags that improve with stimulation
D. disruption in psychosocial environment

29. In treating the above patient, a nurse should 29.____

A. monitor input and output and describe the frequency and precipitating events of any vomiting
B. observe feeding patterns
C. obtain daily weights before breakfast on the same scale and weekly length and head circumferences
D. all of the above

30. If the patient shows progression in development while hospitalized, the nurse should do all of the following EXCEPT 30.____

A. not use primary caregivers
B. monitor the patient's response to care
C. hold, cuddle, and talk to the infant lovingly
D. provide age-appropriate developmental and sensory stimulation

31. If the infant's parents show positive interaction with him, the nurse should NOT 31.____

A. welcome the parents when visiting
B. discourage their participation in the patient's care
C. use anticipatory guidance regarding the patient's capabilities, physical care, and emotional needs
D. all of the above

32. A patient is admitted to the hospital with gross hema-turia and periorbital edema which developed two weeks after a throat infection. A diagnosis of acute glomerulo-nephritis (AGN) is made. 32.____
Which of the following laboratory tests would INITIALLY be done upon admission?

A. Complete blood count
B. Serum electrolyte and chemistry
C. Urine culture and urine for amino acids
D. Blood culture

33. Nutrients stored in the body are drawn upon, in the absence of sufficient food intake, in the following order: 33.____

A. Fats, carbohydrates, water, lactic acid
B. Carbohydrates, water, lactic acid, fats
C. Water, carbohydrates, lactic acid, fats
D. Lactic acid, water, carbohydrates, fats

34. Vitamin B complex deficiency is associated with 34.____

A. beriberi
B. enlargement of the liver
C. pellagra
D. all of the above

35. Roughage is necessary in the diet in order to promote optimal 35.____

A. digestion
B. peristalsis
C. absorption
D. all of the above

KEY (CORRECT ANSWERS)

1.	C	11.	B	21.	C	31.	B
2.	D	12.	D	22.	D	32.	B
3.	D	13.	C	23.	C	33.	C
4.	C	14.	A	24.	C	34.	D
5.	A	15.	D	25.	B	35.	B
6.	B	16.	B	26.	C		
7.	B	17.	D	27.	C		
8.	C	18.	B	28.	C		
9.	D	19.	C	29.	D		
10.	A	20.	A	30.	A		

EXAMINATION SECTION
TEST 1

DIRECTIONS: Each question or incomplete statement is followed by several suggested answers or completions. Select the one that BEST answers the question or completes the statement. *PRINT THE LETTER OF THE CORRECT ANSWER IN THE SPACE AT THE RIGHT.*

1. According to Freudian theory, the ______ functions to encourage a person's tolerance of frustration. 1.____

   A. subconscious
   B. id
   C. ego
   D. superego

2. Which of the following hormones controls the use of glucose by the body's cells? 2.____

   A. Cortisone
   B. Insulin
   C. Adrenal steroids
   D. Thyroxine

3. A client who is receiving lithium carbonate should undergo regular monitoring of 3.____

   A. blood pressure
   B. blood level
   C. weight
   D. urine

4. According to intrapsychic theory, the problem of separation anxiety is MOST likely to occur during the ______ stage. 4.____

   A. latency
   B. oral
   C. anal
   D. phallic

5. A client with adrenal insufficiency is weak and dizzy upon arising in the morning. The MOST likely cause of this is 5.____

   A. lack of sodium
   B. increased intracavity fluid volume
   C. hypertension
   D. hypoglycemic reaction

6. The administration of Anectine prior to electroconvulsive therapy involves the major complication of 6.____

   A. loss of bowel control
   B. inhibition of breathing muscles
   C. memory loss
   D. the bite reflex

7. An infant with congenital hyperthyroidism is at risk for ______ if care is not given immediately. 7.____

   A. thyrotoxicosis
   B. acromegaly
   C. myxedema
   D. mental retardation

8. For which of the following is lithium carbonate used as a control or modifier? 8.____

   A. Manic episode of bipolar disorder
   B. Acute agitation of schizophrenia

C. Agitated phase of paranoia
D. Depressive phase of major depression

9. Which of the following is the cause of acromegaly? 9.____

A. Oversecretion of adrenal steroids
B. Undersecretion of thyroid hormone
C. Oversecretion of growth hormone
D. Undersecretion of testosterone

10. At what approximate age does a person demonstrate the primary emergence of his or her personality? 10.____

A. 6 months
B. 18 months
C. 2 years
D. 8 years

11. Diabetic acidosis is caused by elevated ______ levels in the blood. 11.____

A. lactic acid
B. ketone
C. albumin
D. glucose

12. Which of the following behaviors is MOST likely to be demonstrated by an autistic child? 12.____

A. Lack of response to external stimuli
B. Sad facial expression
C. Irrelevant smiling
D. Rocking and flapping of hands

13. To evaluate the effectiveness of DDAVP in treating diabetes insipidus, which of the following should be monitored? 13.____

A. Blood pressure
B. Intake and output
C. Pulse rate
D. Serum glucose

14. Glucagon 14.____

A. retards glycogenesis
B. causes the release of insulin
C. elevates blood sugar levels
D. improves the storage of glucose

15. Of the following, the clearest evidence of mental illness is when a client 15.____

A. does not seem to be able to complete tasks
B. has difficulty relating to others
C. has little interest in social activities or work
D. encounters frequent periods of high anxiety

16. For a client with insulin-dependent diabetes mellitus, insulin needs will *decrease* when the client 16.____

A. exercises
B. is infected
C. reaches middle age
D. is emotionally stressed

17. The treatment for a client suffering from depression should focus on getting the client to 17.____

A. express anger toward others
B. admit an emotional problem
C. articulate feelings of low self-esteem
D. accept care and comfort willingly

18. A child who is about to undergo surgery to correct a congenital megacolon should be given a preoperative enema of 18.____

A. barium
B. isotonic saline
C. tap water
D. hypertonic phosphate

19. Which of the following is a common side effect associated with the use of Thorazine? 19.____

A. Jaundice
B. Melanocytosis
C. Photosensitivity
D. Excessive thirst

20. Piaget's theory of cognitive development states that at the age of six months, an infant should demonstrate 20.____

A. a sense of time
B. the ability to remember
C. the onset of object permanence
D. coordinated motor responses

21. Which of the following would MOST clearly reveal congenital hip dysplasia in a newborn infant? 21.____

A. Different leg lengths
B. Asymmetrical gluteal folds
C. Limited adduction
D. Skewed leg alignment

22. A client is diagnosed with an organic mental disorder. Which of the following nursing strategies would be MOST helpful to this client? 22.____

A. Providing a diet high in carbohydrates
B. Providing a variety of stimuli to keep the client's interest high
C. Eliminating the need for choices
D. Asking the client for input concerning the nursing care plan

23. Which of the following would be included in the early treatment of diabetic acidosis? 23.____

A. IV fluids
B. Kayexalate
C. Potassium
D. NPH insulin

24. Which level of consciousness BEST represents a person's feelings and attitudes? 24.____

A. Conscious
B. Unconscious
C. Preconscious
D. Foreconscious

25. What is the MOST common cause of diabetic ketoacidosis? 25.____

A. Inadequate fluid intake
B. Psychological stress
C. Elevated insulin level
D. Infection

KEY (CORRECT ANSWERS)

1. C
2. C
3. B
4. B
5. D
6. B
7. D
8. A
9. C
10. C
11. B
12. D
13. B
14. C
15. B
16. A
17. A
18. B
19. C
20. C
21. B
22. C
23. A
24. B
25. D

TEST 2

DIRECTIONS: Each question or incomplete statement is followed by several suggested answers or completions. Select the one that BEST answers the question or completes the statement. *PRINT THE LETTER OF THE CORRECT ANSWER IN THE SPACE AT THE RIGHT.*

1. A client with an anxiety disorder is likely to handle the anxiety in each of the following ways EXCEPT 1.____

   A. projecting it onto nonthreatening objects
   B. converting it into a physical symptom
   C. demonstrating regressive behavior
   D. acting out with antisocial behavior

2. What type of diet is recommended for a client with Graves' disease? 2.____

   A. High roughage
   B. Low sodium
   C. Liquid
   D. High-calorie

3. Which of the following is the cause of primary degenerative dementia? 3.____

   A. Anatomic brain changes
   B. Atrophy of the frontal lobes
   C. An extended history of malnutrition
   D. Excessive use of narcotics

4. Which of the following blood gas results would indicate diabetic acidosis? 4.____

   A. Reduced HCO_3
   B. Elevated pH
   C. Reduced PO_2
   D. Elevated PCO_2

5. The primary difference between a psychophysiologic disorder and a somatoform disorder is that a 5.____

   A. psychophysiologic disorder involves an actual change in tissues
   B. somatoform disorder is caused by emotions
   C. psychophysiologic disorder restricts the client's activities
   D. somatoform disorder is accompanied by a feeling of illness

6. Which of the following is MOST likely to be a complication following the insertion of a ventriculoperitoneal shunt in a child with communicating hydrocephalus? 6.____

   A. Violent tremors
   B. Distended abdomen
   C. Yellowish discharge from shunt
   D. Fever

7. Each of the following is a common physiological response to anxiety EXCEPT 7.____

   A. respiratory constriction
   B. dilated pupils
   C. hyperglycemia
   D. increased pulse rate

8. It is MOST important for a nurse to monitor a client suffering from alcohol and cirrhosis for 8.____

A. gastric pain
B. blood in the stool
C. dizziness
D. constipation

9. To encourage a withdrawn and noncommunicative client to talk, the BEST nursing plan would include the attempt to 9.____

A. ask the client to describe feelings
B. ask simply-phrased questions that require yes or no answers
C. join the client in an activity that the client enjoys
D. concentrate on subjects that are nonthreatening

10. What is the function of glucose in a cell? 10.____

A. Energy extraction
B. Protein synthesis
C. Cellular respiration
D. Genetic coding

11. Which of the following treatments would be included in a plan for a client with severe and intractable depression and suicidal tendency? 11.____

A. High doses of tranquilizers
B. Electroconvulsive therapy
C. Nondirective psychotherapy
D. Thorazine

12. A *decrease* in the anterior pituitary secretion of ACTH would be caused by 12.____

A. ketosis
B. a *decrease* in the blood concentration of adrenal steroids
C. an *increase* in the blood concentration of cortisol
D. acidosis

13. A client is experiencing a phase of extreme elation and hyperactivity. Which of the following nursing interventions would BEST meet the client's nutritional needs? 13.____

A. Assuming that the client will eat when hungry
B. Firmly suggesting that the client sit and eat the meal that has been prepared
C. Inducing an IV feeding to insure that the client is properly nourished
D. Giving the client frequent high-calorie feedings that the client can feed to herself

14. Which of the following would be experienced by a client with acute cholecystitis accompanied by biliary colic? 14.____

A. Melena
B. Lipid intolerance
C. Diarrhea
D. Pain in lower left quadrant

15. Which of the following must be monitored especially closely following a hypophysectomy? 15.____

A. Motor reflexes
B. Urinary output
C. Intracranial pressure
D. Respiration

16. Which of the following would MOST accurately characterize the personality of a client with obsessive-compulsive personality disorder? 16.____

A. Deep depression
B. Indecisiveness and doubt
C. Rapid mood swings
D. Detailed delusions

17. Which of the following symptoms would MOST likely be revealed during an assessment of a client with Cushing's syndrome? 17.____

A. Dehydration
B. Migraine headaches
C. Menorrhagia
D. Hypertension

18. Most commonly, the behavior of a client with schizophrenia can be described as 18.____

A. euphoric
B. angry and hostile
C. flat and apathetic
D. depressed

19. Which of the following medications would be used to treat a child with cystic fibrosis? 19.____

A. Antimetabolite
B. Pancreatic enzymes
C. Fat-soluble vitamins
D. Aerosol mists

20. Which of the following would NOT be a helpful component of a nursing care plan for a severely depressed client? 20.____

A. Short-term projects
B. Client participation in activity planning
C. Repetitive activities
D. Simple instructions to be followed

21. A client with Addison's disease is experiencing hypotension. Most likely, this involves a disturbance in the production of 21.____

A. mineralocorticoids
B. proteins
C. glucocorticoids
D. insulin

22. Which of the following medications would be used to counter an overdose of narcotics? 22.____

A. Methadone
B. Thorazine
C. Benzedrine
D. Narcan

23. Prior to a serum glucose test, a client with Type II diabetes mellitus should 23.____

A. have a clear liquid breakfast
B. take prescribed medications
C. void the bladder
D. avoid food and fluids

24. Which of the following is the BEST description of a somatoform disorder? A(n) 24.____

A. conscious defense against stress
B. sublimation of stress
C. psychological defense against anxiety
D. unconscious means of controlling conflict

25. Which of the following tests is conducted to detect PKU in infant children? 25.____

A. OCT
B. Phenistix test
C. BUN
D. Guthrie blood test

KEY (CORRECT ANSWERS)

1. D
2. D
3. B
4. A
5. A

6. D
7. A
8. B
9. D
10. A

11. B
12. C
13. D
14. B
15. C

16. B
17. B
18. C
19. B
20. B

21. A
22. D
23. D
24. D
25. D

TEST 3

DIRECTIONS: Each question or incomplete statement is followed by several suggested answers or completions. Select the one that BEST answers the question or completes the statement. *PRINT THE LETTER OF THE CORRECT ANSWER IN THE SPACE AT THE RIGHT.*

1. A client recently admitted to an alcohol detoxification unit would probably exhibit each of the following EXCEPT 1.____

   A. hypertension B. nausea
   C. hyperactivity D. loss of appetite

2. Prior to an adrenalectomy, the client should 2.____

   A. increase fluid intake
   B. receive steroids
   C. have all medication withheld for 48 hours
   D. be placed on a high-protein diet

3. A client with an antisocial personality disorder 3.____

   A. learns quickly through experience and punishment
   B. is generally unable to defer gratification
   C. often masks his disorder by articulate communication
   D. suffers from a high level of anxiety

4. Which of the following is a defense mechanism that helps an individual channel unacceptable desires into socially approved behavior? 4.____

   A. Regression B. Denial
   C. Conversion D. Sublimation

5. Which of the following would NOT be a likely result of a laboratory test performed on a client suffering from diabetic ketoacidosis? 5.____

   A. Low CO_2 B. Increased acidity
   C. High bicarbonate D. Increased blood sugar

6. Following an adrenalectomy, a client is MOST likely to exhibit the symptoms of 6.____

   A. sodium retention B. dehydration
   C. hypotension D. increased urinary output

7. It is MOST important for a nurse to ______ when attempting to resolve a crisis situation with a client. 7.____

   A. encourage socialization
   B. meet all of the client's dependency needs
   C. nurture the client's ego strengths
   D. introduce the client to a therapy group

8. Which of the following is NOT a typical indication of a hypoglycemic reaction to insulin? 8.____

   A. Paleness B. Excessive thirst
   C. Tremors D. Perspiration

9. A client is admitted to the hospital with a diagnosis of conversion disorder. The nurse should expect the client's attitude toward his physical symptoms to be one of 9.____

A. hysteria
B. indifference
C. anger
D. great sadness

10. Along with vitamin D, the regulatory agent that controls the overall calcium balance in the body is 10.____

A. parathyroid hormone
B. growth hormone
C. thyroid hormone
D. ACTH

11. A client is admitted to the hospital with Wernicke's encephalopathy caused by chronic alcoholism. The client's initial treatment would include 11.____

A. an increase in fluid intake
B. IM injection of thiamine
C. administration of an anti-opiate
D. administration of paraldehyde

12. Each of the following is a defect commonly associated with tetralogy of Fallot EXCEPT 12.____

A. pulmonary artery stenosis
B. mitral valve stenosis
C. right ventricular hypertrophy
D. overriding aorta

13. Which of the following statements, spoken to a nurse by a patient diagnosed with Alzheimer's disease, would indicate a need to accomplish Erikson's developmental task of ego integrity versus despair? 13.____

A. I don't understand why I have to go through this.
B. Please leave me alone.
C. I can take care of myself.
D. I am useless to everyone now.

14. The purpose of administering Mycifradin to a client with liver disease is to 14.____

A. increase the urea digestive activity of enteric bacteria
B. protect the liver from bacteria
C. reduce ammonia-forming bacteria in the intestinal tract
D. aid the digestion of complex proteins

15. Emotionally disturbed children 15.____

A. seem unresponsive to their environment
B. respond equally to all stimuli
C. respond violently to most stimuli
D. are immersed in their environment to the point of distraction

16. A client exhibiting cold intolerance may have 16.____

A. increased levels of CO_2
B. decreased blood pH

C. insufficient bile salts
D. decreased levels of T_3 and T_4

17. The part of the psyche that develops from internalizing the concepts of parents and other significant relations is the 17.____

A. foreconscious
B. id
C. ego
D. superego

18. Which of the following is NOT a typical sign of hypo-kalemia? 18.____

A. Weakness
B. Abdominal distention
C. Edema
D. Apathy

19. Which of the following might be experienced by a person who makes an abrupt withdrawal from habitual use of barbiturates? 19.____

A. Gastric bleeding
B. Cardiac arrhythmia
C. Convulsions
D. Ataxia

20. Which of the following would be observed in a toddler with cyanotic congenital heart disease? 20.____

A. Orthopnea
B. Blotchy skin
C. Increased hematocrit
D. Pitting edema

21. A delusional client is admitted for psychiatric treatment after harming a close relative. In talking about the incident, the client refers to herself in the third person. This is an example of the defense mechanism of 21.____

A. conversion
B. transference
C. dissociation
D. displacement

22. Which of the following is the clearest indication of diabetes insipidus? 22.____

A. Elevated blood glucose
B. Increased blood pressure
C. Decreased urinary specific gravity
D. Increased BUN

23. Which of the following is the MOST common cause of functional mental illness? 23.____

A. Infection
B. Chemical imbalance
C. Social environment
D. Genes

24. Which gland regulates the rate of oxygenation in the body's cells? 24.____

A. Thyroid
B. Adrenal
C. Thalamus
D. Pituitary

25. Which of the following is NOT thought to be a significant formative component of personality? 25.____

A. Cultural setting
B. Genetic background
C. Psychologic development
D. Biologic constitution

KEY (CORRECT ANSWERS)

1. C
2. B
3. B
4. D
5. C

6. C
7. C
8. B
9. B
10. A

11. B
12. B
13. D
14. C
15. A

16. D
17. D
18. C
19. C
20. C

21. C
22. B
23. C
24. A
25. B

TEST 4

DIRECTIONS: Each question or incomplete statement is followed by several suggested answers or completions. Select the one that BEST answers the question or completes the statement. *PRINT THE LETTER OF THE CORRECT ANSWER IN THE SPACE AT THE RIGHT.*

1. The preservation of sodium in the body's cells is accomplished by the hormone 1.____

   A. parathyroid hormone
   B. thyrocalcitonin
   C. aldosterone
   D. insulin

2. Which of the following behaviors would be LEAST likely to be demonstrated by a client with an organic mental disorder? 2.____

   A. An inclination to ignore the present circumstances while dwelling in the past
   B. A steadfast resistance to change
   C. The inability to focus on new interests
   D. A fixation on personal appearance and hygiene

3. Which of the following is a complication associated with hyperparathyroidism? 3.____

   A. Bone destruction
   B. Graves' disease
   C. Hypotension
   D. Tetany

4. Which of the following interventions should be undertaken to prevent thrombus formation in a client with sickle-cell anemia? 4.____

   A. Administer heparin or other anticoagulants
   B. Encourage exercise
   C. Maintain a high-roughage diet
   D. Increase oral fluid intake

5. A client with an obsessive-compulsive personality disorder will MOST likely react with ______ if he is interrupted in the performance of a ritual. 5.____

   A. hostility
   B. indifference
   C. confusion
   D. withdrawal

6. Which of the following would be experienced by a patient in a diabetic coma, but not by a patient in an HHNK coma? 6.____

   A. Kussmaul respirations
   B. Glycosuria
   C. Fluid loss
   D. Elevated blood glucose

7. Which of the following daily patterns tends to work best with clients who are depressed? 7.____

   A. Numerous sensory stimuli
   B. A simple daily schedule
   C. Removing the need for complicated decisions
   D. Multiple and varied activities

8. Glucocorticoids are secreted by the 8.____

   A. hypophysis cerebri
   B. adrenal glands
   C. thyroid
   D. pancreas

9. Prior to beginning lithium carbonate therapy, a client should undergo 9.____

A. fluid and electrolyte evaluation
B. renal evaluation
C. psychomotor
D. BUN evaluation

10. Which of the following is the result of an underproduction of thyroxin? 10.____

A. Acromegaly
B. Cushing's disease
C. Myxedema
D. Addison's disease

11. Which of the following is a common side effect of the major tranquilizers? 11.____

A. Tremors
B. Diaphoresis
C. Jaundice
D. Photosensitivity

12. Each of the following is likely to be revealed during the assessment of a client with hyperthyroidism EXCEPT 12.____

A. weight loss
B. increased appetite
C. constipation
D. nervousness

13. Severe emotional disturbances are often treated with tranquilizers to 13.____

A. prevent complications
B. make the client less dangerous to himself and others
C. improve the client's mood
D. make the client more receptive to psychotherapy

14. Which of the following symptoms would cause a nurse to stop giving Thorazine to a client? 14.____

A. Uncoordinated movements
B. Jaundice
C. Withdrawal
D. Tremors

15. What is the MOST likely cause of ascites in a patient with cirrhosis? 15.____

A. Inhibited portal venous return
B. Undersecretion of bile salts
C. Gastric bleeding
D. Overproduction of serum albumin

16. The defense mechanism used by clients who express anxiety through physical symptoms can BEST be described as 16.____

A. psychosomatic
B. regressive
C. psychoneurotic
D. dissociative

17. A 42-year-old client is admitted to the hospital with a diagnosis of Addison's disease. She is weak, hypotensive, and has low sodium and high potassium levels.
The focus of the client's therapy should be 17.____

A. lowering the level of eosiniphils
B. restoring electrolyte balance
C. increasing carbohydrate intake
D. increasing lymph

18. A client who has been hospitalized for major depression has recently begun to receive Parnate. It is important that the nurse explain to the client that the use of this drug 18.____

A. typically causes extreme photosensitivity
B. may cause drowsiness
C. increases the heart rate
D. involves dietary restrictions

19. The MOST frequent cause of Cushing's syndrome is 19.____

A. hyperplasia of pituitary
B. hyperplasia of adrenal cortex
C. decreased adrenocortical hormones
D. insufficient production of ACTH

20. A group setting is particularly conducive to therapy because it 20.____

A. takes the focus off the individual client
B. forces clients to notice similarities with others
C. establishes a learning environment
D. encourages individual relationships

21. What is the purpose of installing a T-tube after a cholecystectomy? 21.____

A. Draining bile from the cystic duct
B. Protecting the common bile duct
C. Preventing infection
D. Providing a port for cholangiogram dye

22. A nurse notices that a socially agressive elderly client, who has been receiving Thorazine for several months, is sitting rigidly in a chair. What other adverse effects of the drug should the nurse watch for? 22.____

A. Tremors
B. Slurred speech
C. Excessive salivation
D. Withdrawal

23. For what reason is an infant born with a cleft palate prone to infection? 23.____

A. Mouth breathing
B. Leakage of nasal mucus
C. Poor nutrition from feeding disturbances
D. Poor circulation in defective locus

24. Which of the following is a defense mechanism in which emotional conflicts are expressed through sensorimotor or somatic disability? 24.____

A. Dissociation
B. Conversion
C. Displacement
D. Regression

25. For the emergency treatment of ketoacidosis, what type of insulin should be administered? 25.____

A. Zinc suspension
B. NPH insulin
C. Protamine zinc suspension
D. Regular insulin injection

KEY (CORRECT ANSWERS)

1.	C	11.	A
2.	D	12.	C
3.	A	13.	D
4.	D	14.	B
5.	A	15.	A
6.	A	16.	C
7.	B	17.	B
8.	D	18.	D
9.	B	19.	B
10.	C	20.	C

21. B
22. A
23. A
24. B
25. D

EXAMINATION SECTION

TEST 1

DIRECTIONS: Refer to the pictures indicated (at the end of Test 2, page 8) and use the patient information provided to answer the questions that follow. Each question or incomplete statement is followed by several suggested answers or completions. Select the one that BEST answers the question or completes the statement. *PRINT THE LETTER OF THE CORRECT ANSWER IN THE SPACE AT THE RIGHT.*

Refer to photo #1 and the patient information below to answer Questions 1 through 6:

Demographics: 3-year-old male
Chief complaint: Blepharospasm, epiphora, photophobia
Secondary complaints/symptoms: none
Patient's ocular history: Large cornea, complaints present from birth onwards
Patient's medical history: not significant
Medications taken by patient: Nasal decongestants, antihistamines
Family ocular history: Mother and father normal
Family medical history: not significant
Clinical findings: Both eyes – large cornea, corneal edema - positive
Pupils: normal size and normal reaction
Fundus: C:D::0.5:1, IOP – 22 mmHg by NCT

1. Which of the following is the most likely diagnosis? 1.______
   A. Congenital cataract
   B. Buphthalmos
   C. Megalocornea
   D. Blunt trauma in both eyes

2. What is the mode of inheritance of this disease? 2.______
   A. Autosomal recessive
   B. Autosomal dominant
   C. Sporadic
   D. Sex linked disease

3. The disease usually affects 3.______
   A. boys more than girls
   B. girls more than boys
   C. both girls and boys equally
   D. none of the above

4. What are the other clinical features of this condition that would contribute to the diagnosis? 4.______
   A. Deep anterior chamber
   B. Subluxated lens
   C. Haab's striae
   D. All of the above

5. Which feature does not differentiate megalocornea from buphthalmos? 5.______
   A. Normal fundus
   B. Normal anterior chamber
   C. Normal intraocular pressure
   D. Bilateral

6. Which is not included in the diagnosis of buphthalmos? 6.______
   A. IOP of 21 mmHg under halothane anesthesia
   B. Corneal diameter above 12 mm in first year of life
   C. High insertion of iris at or above the scleral spur
   D. Vertical tears in the descemet's membrane

Refer to photo #2 and the patient information below to answer Questions 7 through 12:

Demographics: 58-year-old male farmer
Chief complaint: OD – Pain, diminution of vision, blepharospasm; OS – normal
Secondary complaints/symptoms: none
Patient's ocular history: History of injury with vegetable matter in right eye – two days
Patient's medical history: Diabetes
Medications taken by patient: None
Family ocular history: None
Family medical history: Diabetes
Clinical findings: BCVA OD – 6/36, OS – 6/9; OD – Corneal ulcer
Pupils: normal size and normal reaction; anterior chamber – hypopyon; OS – normal
Slit lamp examination: Lids normal, conjunctiva congested, circumcorneal congestion, cornea—ulcer, anterior chamber—hypopyon, lens normal, vitreous—appears normal; OS – normal
IOP: OD – digitally normal, slightly more than OS
Fundus: OD – not clearly visible but appears normal; OS – normal

7. What is the most likely diagnosis of this condition? 7.______
   A. Corneal epithelial defect
   B. Bacterial corneal ulcer
   C. Viral corneal ulcer
   D. Fungal corneal ulcer

8. What nature of hypopyon is expected in this condition? 8.______
   A. Freely mobile B. Immobile
   C. Watery D. None of the above

9. Which is the most confirmatory test for this condition? 9.______
   A. Slit lamp examination
   B. Ultrasonography
   C. Corneal smear followed by KOH stain
   D. Corneal smear followed by KOH stain and culture

10. What are the stains useful in diagnosing acanthamoeba corneal ulcer? 10.______
    A. Calcoflour white stain
    B. Methylene blue
    C. Gram's stain
    D. Ziehl Neelson stain

11. Which is not a feature of pseudomonas corneal ulcer? 11.______
    A. Yellowish-green purulent material
    B. Can spread from fluorescein solution
    C. Rapid progression leading to perforation
    D. Immobile hypopyon

12. Which is not true of acanthamoeba ulcer? 12.______
    A. Radial keratoneuritis
    B. Common in contact lens wearers
    C. Can be treated with antibacterials
    D. Pain is severe and out of proportion

Refer to photo #3 and the patient information below to answer Questions 13 through 22:

Demographics: 14-year-old male
Chief complaint: Sudden diminution of vision – one day
Secondary complaints/symptoms: none
Patient's ocular history: Blunt trauma with a stone in left eye – one day
Patient's medical history: None
Medications taken by patient: None
Patient's allergic history: None
Family ocular history: None
Family medical history: None
Clinical findings: BCVA OD – 6/5 and normal anterior and posterior segment; OS – 6/36, slight afferent pupillary defect
Slit lamp examination: OD – lids, conjunctiva, cornea and anterior segment normal, vitreous normal; OS – slight vitreous haze
IOP: OD – normal, OS – slightly low
Fundus: OD – normal, OS – superior retinal detachment, optic disc normal, fovea normal

13. What is the most important examination to be done to make a diagnosis in this patient? 13.______
    A. Direct ophthalmoscopy
    B. Distant direct ophthalmoscopy
    C. Indirect ophthalmoscopy
    D. Slit lamp examination

14. What is the investigation modality you would order to confirm the diagnosis? 14.______
    A. USG A scan
    B. USG B scan
    C. CT scan
    D. MRI scan

15. What is the likely clinical course of this condition if it is left untreated? 15.______
    A. Progress to total retinal detachment
    B. Remains stationary
    C. Retina would spontaneously attach
    D. Retinal fibrosis

16. The underlying cause of retinal detachment due to trauma with a stone is 16.______
    A. exudative
    B. tractional
    C. rhegmatogenous
    D. all of the above

17. Disturbance to vitreous at which site is most likely to cause retinal detachment? 17.______
    A. Vitreous base
    B. Around the peripheral retinal blood vessels
    C. Around fovea
    D. Posterior border of lattice degeneration

18. Which of the peripheral retinal changes is least likely to cause the formation of retinal breaks? 18.______
    A. Lattice degeneration
    B. Snail track degeneration
    C. White with pressure
    D. White without pressure

19. Which of these factors does not predispose the myopic eyes to develop retinal detachment? 19.______
    A. Lattice degeneration
    B. Diffuse chorioretinal atrophy
    C. Liquefied vitreous
    D. More axial length than normal eyes

20. The exudative retinal detachment is found in all EXCEPT 20.______
    A. myopia
    B. Vogt Koyanagi Harada disease
    C. panretinal photocoagulation
    D. pregnancy

21. Longstanding retinal detachment has which of the following features? 21.______
    A. Retinal thinning
    B. Secondary intraretinal cysts
    C. Subretinal demarcation lines
    D. All of the above

22. Which is not a feature of tractional retinal detachment? 22.______
    A. Breaks
    B. Concave configuration
    C. Reduced mobility of retina
    D. Found in diabetes

Refer to photo #8 and the patient information below to answer Questions 23 through 26:

Demographics: 30-year-old female
Chief complaint: Erythematous skin eruptions all over the body, redness of eyes with watering following intake of systemic sulphonamide for upper respiratory infection
Secondary complaints/symptoms: Dryness and foreign body sensation in eyes
Patient's ocular history: Not significant
Patient's medical history: Nil
Medications taken by patient: Sulphonamide systemically
Patient's allergic history: Nil
Family ocular history: Not significant
Family medical history: Father has diabetes
Clinical findings: BCVA 6/12 OD:OS
Pupils: Both eyes normal size and normal reaction
Slit lamp examination: Mucopurulent conjunctivitis with inflame papillae, ischaemic conjunctiva with white-yellow membranes, dryness of eyes with decreased tear film breakup time
Fundus: Appears normal

23. What is the most probable diagnosis of this condition? 23.______
    A. Hemorrhagic conjunctivitis
    B. Viral conjunctivitis
    C. Stevens Johnson syndrome
    D. Trachoma

24. What are the agents which can cause this disease condition? 24.______
    A. Herpes simplex
    B. Mycoplasma pneumoniae
    C. Mumps
    D. All of the above

25. The ocular clinical features not found in this disease are 25.______
    A. cataract
    B. metaplastic eyelashes
    C. cicatricial entropion
    D. keratinization of conjunctiva

26. The systemic features of this disease include all EXCEPT 26.______
    A. erythematous popular eruption
    B. fever and malaise
    C. liver enlargement
    D. involvement of mucus membrane of nose and mouth

KEY (CORRECT ANSWERS)

1. B	11. D	21. D
2. A	12. C	22. A
3. A	13. C	23. C
4. D	14. B	24. D
5. D	15. A	25. A
6. D	16. C	26. C
7. D	17. A	
8. B	18. C	
9. D	19. D	
10. A	20. A	

TEST 2

DIRECTIONS: Refer to the picture indicated and use the patient information provided to answer the questions that follow. Each question or incomplete statement is followed by several suggested answers or completions. Select the one that BEST answers the question or completes the statement. *PRINT THE LETTER OF THE CORRECT ANSWER IN THE SPACE AT THE RIGHT.*

Refer to photo #4 and the patient information below to answer Questions 1 through 6:

Demographics: 60-year-old female, teacher
Chief complaint: Diminution of vision in both eyes – two months
Secondary complaints/symptoms: Dryness of both eyes with foreign body sensation
Patient's ocular history: Last examination done two years ago, patient wears reading glasses
Patient's medical history: Diabetes for last 20 years
Medications taken by patient: Topical artificial tears in both eyes
Family ocular history: Both mother and father had cataract surgery in both eyes
Family medical history: Father had diabetes
Clinical findings: Best corrected visual acuity – 6/24 both eyes
Pupils: normal size and normal reaction
Slit lamp: Lids, conjunctiva, cornea are normal and anterior chamber and iris are normal; early senile cataract in both eyes and vitreous is normal
IOP: 18 mmHg in both eyes by applanation tonometry
Fundus: C:D::0.3, foveal reflex – sharp, background diabetic retinopathy both eyes

1. What is the most likely cause of diminution of vision? 1.______
    A. Refractive error in both eyes
    B. Macular edema
    C. Background diabetic retinopathy
    D. Corneal edema

2. Which test is most appropriate to measure the effect of diabetic retinopathy on vision? 2.______
    A. Fluorescein angiography
    B. Slit lamp examination
    C. Indocyanine green angiography
    D. Indirect ophthalmoscopy

3. Which test would you not like to advise to see the control of blood sugar in this patient? 3.______
    A. Glycosylated hemoglobin
    B. Microalbuminuria
    C. Blood sugar fasting and post prandial
    D. MRI scan of head and orbit

4. The stage of diabetic retinopathy which this patient has is 4.______
   A. background B. preproliferative
   C. proliferative D. none of the above

5. All of the following are features of background diabetic retinopathy EXCEPT 5.______
   A. microaneurysms B. hard exudates
   C. venous beading D. central retinal vein occlusion

6. Proliferative diabetic retinopathy includes all of the following features EXCEPT 6.______
   A. central retinal artery occlusion
   B. neovascularisation disc
   C. neovascularisation in peripheral fundus
   D. vitreous hemorrhage

Refer to photo #5 and the patient information below to answer Questions 7 through 9:

Demographics: 40-year-old female
Chief complaint: Redness in both eyes – two days
Secondary complaints/symptoms: None
Patient's ocular history: Not significant, wears reading glasses
Patient's medical history: Not significant
Medications taken by patient: Nil
Family ocular history: Both mother and father had cataract
Family medical history: Not significant
Clinical findings: BCVA – 20/20 OD:OS
Pupils: Both eyes normal size and normal reaction
Slit lamp: Bilateral conjunctival congestion, profuse watery discharge, lid oedema, sobconjunctival hemorrhage, open anterior chamber angles
IOP: OD=OS=18 mmHg by non-contact tonometry
Fundus: Both eyes within normal limits

7. What is the most likely diagnosis for this patient? 7.______
   A. Acute attack of open angle glaucoma
   B. Acute attack of angle closure glaucoma
   C. Viral keratitis
   D. Acute hemorrhagic conjunctivitis

8. Which of the following tests would be most helpful in confirming the diagnosis? 8.______
   A. Corneal scrapings B. 30-2 field charting
   C. Ultrasonography D. Clinical examination only

9. Which is the most likely course of this disease? 9.______
   A. Resolves spontaneously
   B. Progresses to involve the cornea
   C. Needs antivirals for its full resolution
   D. Can cause panophthalmitis

Refer to photo #6 and the patient information below to answer Questions 10 through 14:

Demographics: 50-year-old male, farmer
Chief complaint: Itching in both eyes
Secondary complaints/symptoms: Foreign body sensation due to rubbing of eyelashes
Patient's ocular history: Similar complaint in the past
Patient's medical history: Not significant
Medications taken by patient: 20% sulphacetamide eye drops four times a day
Patient's allergic history: Nil
Family ocular history: All family members had similar complaint
Family medical history: Not significant
Clinical findings: BCVA – 6/12 OD:OS
Pupils: Both eyes normal size and normal reaction
Slit lamp: Scarring on the upper tarsal conjunctiva of both eyes
IOP: OD=OS=16 mmHg by applanation tonometry
Fundus: Both eyes within normal limits

10. What is the most probable diagnosis of this condition? 10.______
   A. Follicular conjunctivitis
   B. Trachoma
   C. Pseudomembranous conjunctivitis
   D. Membranous conjunctivitis

11. Which feature is considered to be pathognomic for diagnosis of this condition? 11.______
   A. Conjunctival congestion
   B. Marginal keratitis
   C. Follicles and papillae
   D. Entropion of both upper lids

12. What is the most natural course of this disease? 12.______
   A. Acute inflammation in first decade of life and late sequelae appear after many years
   B. Recurrent corneal ulceration
   C. Recurrent blepharitis
   D. Recurrent attacks of acute dacryocystitis

13. The causative organism of this disease is 13.______
    - A. Chlamydia trachomatis
    - B. hemophilus aegyptius
    - C. gonococcus
    - D. pseudomonas

14. Which is not a sequela of this disease condition? 14.______
    - A. Ptosis
    - B. Entropion
    - C. Dry eyes
    - D. Extraocular muscle paralysis

Refer to photo #7 and the patient information below to answer Questions 15 through 17:

Demographics: 5-year-old boy
Chief complaint: Severe itching and redness of both eyes, watering both eyes; all complaints more during spring
Secondary complaints/symptoms: None
Patient's ocular history: Recurrent
Patient's medical history: Not significant
Medications taken by patient: Sodium cromoglycate 2% eye drops four times a day
Patient's allergic history: Seasonal rhinitis
Family ocular history: Elder brother had similar complaints
Family medical history: Not significant
Clinical findings: BCVA – 20/20 OD:OS
Pupils: Both eyes normal size and normal reaction
Slit lamp: Diffuse papillary hyperplasia on superior tarsus, large papillae having flat-topped "cobblestone" appearance, "trantas" dots on the superior limbus

15. What is the most likely diagnosis of this condition? 15.______
    - A. Trachoma
    - B. Follicular conjunctivitis
    - C. Vernal conjunctivitis
    - D. Viral conjunctivitis

16. The corneal signs in this condition are 16.______
    - A. punctate epithelial keratitis
    - B. subepithelial scarring
    - C. pseudogerontoxon
    - D. all of the above

17. The constant clinical features of the above condition include all EXCEPT 17.______
    - A. bilateral
    - B. seasonal
    - C. recurrent
    - D. boys are involved

Refer to photo #9 and the patient information below to answer Questions 18 through 22:

Demographics: 50-year-old male, farmer
Chief complaint: Redness of right eye with sheath of conjunctiva growing onto cornea
Secondary complaints/symptoms: Redness and watering of both eyes
Patient's ocular history: Nil
Patient's medical history: Not significant
Medications taken by patient: Topical antiallergics
Patient's allergic history: Nil
Family ocular history: Not significant
Family medical history: Both parents are hypertensive
Clinical findings: BCVA – 6/9 OD:OS
Pupils: Both eyes normal size and normal reaction
Slit lamp: Wing-like extension of conjunctiva over the cornea in nasal quadrant
IOP: OD=OS=16 mmHg by applanation tonometry
Fundus: Both eyes within normal limits

18. What is the most likely diagnosis of this condition? 18.______
    A. Pterygium
    B. Phylctenular conjunctivitis
    C. Pinguecula
    D. Episceritis

19. The predisposing factors for appearance of this condition are all of the following EXCEPT 19.______
    A. hot climate
    B. exposure to sun
    C. high refractive error
    D. chronic dryness

20. The slit lamp examination of this feature shows 20.______
    A. Haab's striae
    B. Stocker's line
    C. folds in Descemet's membrane
    D. Fleischer's ring

21. The ocular symptoms include all of the following EXCEPT 21.______
    A. redness of conjunctiva
    B. wing-like extension of conjunctiva
    C. corneal opacities
    D. cataract

22. The most common site of occurrence of this lesion is 22.______
    A. nasal quadrant
    B. temporal
    C. superior
    D. inferior

Refer to photo #10 and the patient information below to answer Questions 23 through 26:

Demographics: 15-year-old male
Chief complaint: Severe foreign body sensation, and diminution of vision in right eye – three days; redness in right eye
Secondary complaints/symptoms: Pain in right eye
Patient's ocular history: Similar complaint in the past
Patient's medical history: Not significant
Medications taken by patient: Nature not known
Patient's allergic history: Nil
Family ocular history: Not significant
Family medical history: Nil
Clinical findings: BCVA – OD 6/36, OS 6/9
Pupils: Both eyes normal size and normal reaction
Slit lamp: OD – dendritic lesion on cornea stained with rose Bengal circumcorneal congestion, stromal opacities, endothelium normal, no uveitis, OS normal
Fundus: Appears normal in both eyes

23. The most likely diagnosis of this condition is __________ keratitis. 23.______
    A. bacterial
    B. fungal
    C. viral
    D. acanthamoeba

24. The ocular lesions that can occur in this condition are 24.______
    A. geographical ulcers
    B. endothelitis
    C. disciform keratitis
    D. all of the above

25. Other causes of dendritic ulceration of the cornea include all of the following EXCEPT 25.______
    A. herpes zoster keratitis
    B. Thygeson's superficial punctate keratitis
    C. healing corneal abrasion
    D. ringworm infection

26. The diagnostic conditions of this disease condition include all of the following EXCEPT 26.______
    A. recurrent
    B. involvement of females
    C. immunosuppression
    D. bilateral

KEY (CORRECT ANSWERS)

1. B	11. C	21. D
2. A	12. A	22. A
3. D	13. A	23. C
4. A	14. D	24. D
5. D	15. C	25. D
6. A	16. D	26. B
7. D	17. D	
8. D	18. A	
9. A	19. C	
10. B	20. B	

8 (#2)

1

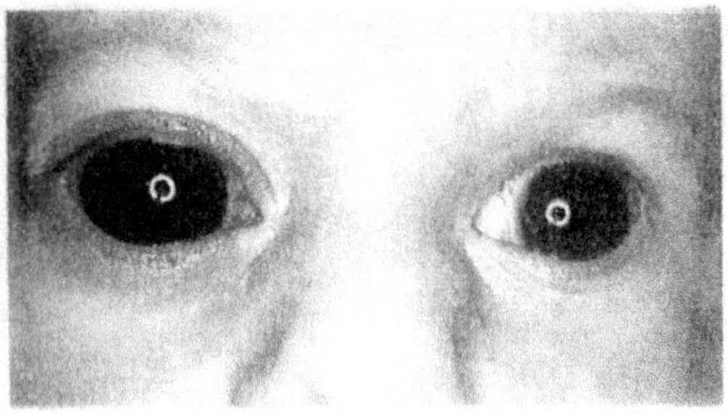

2

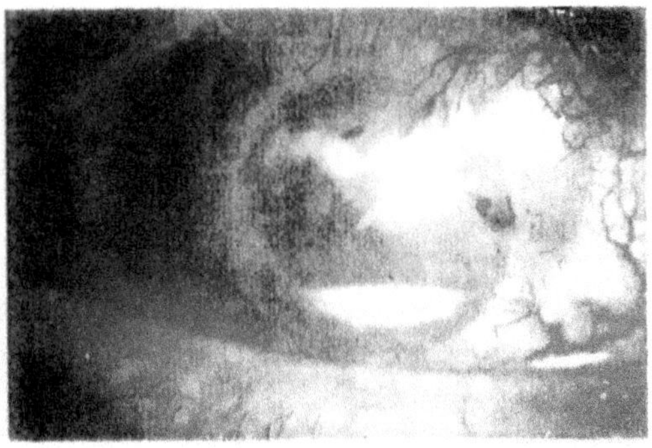

3

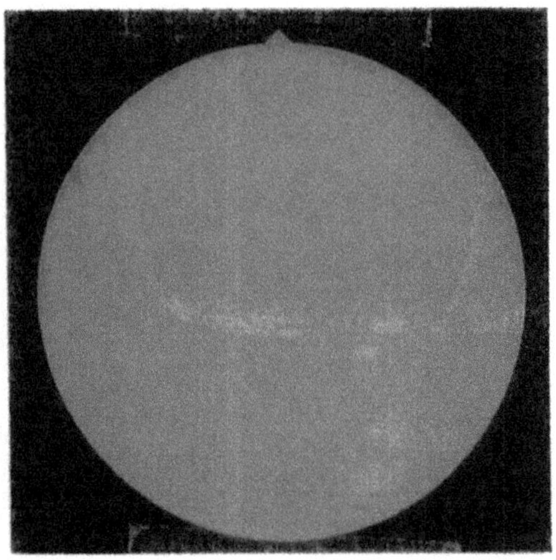

4

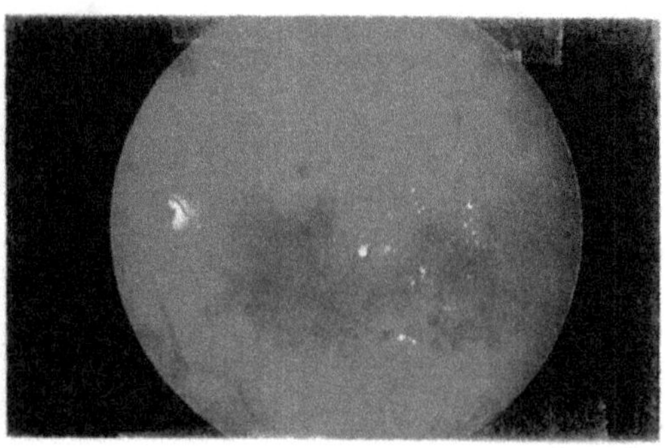

5

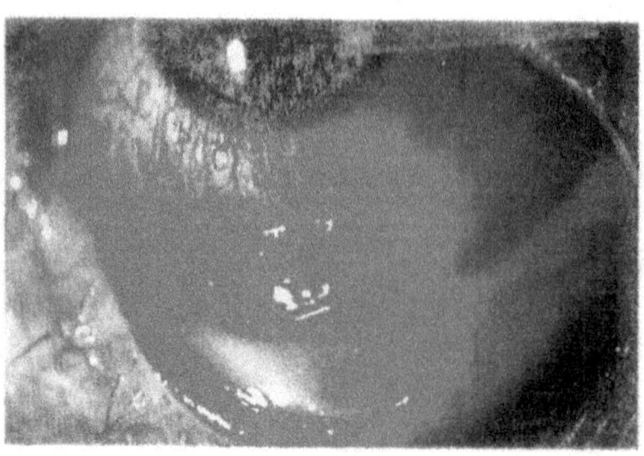

6

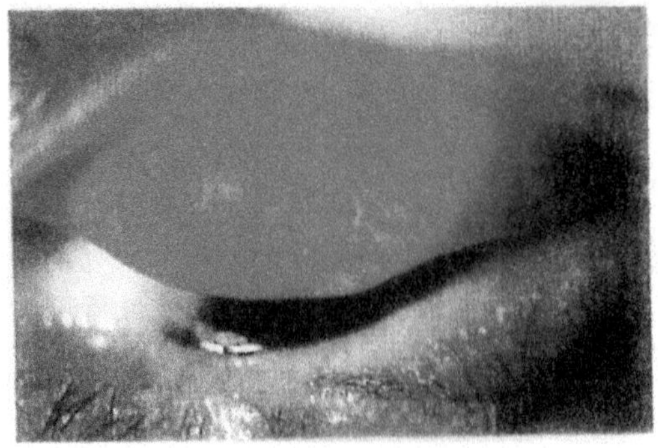

7

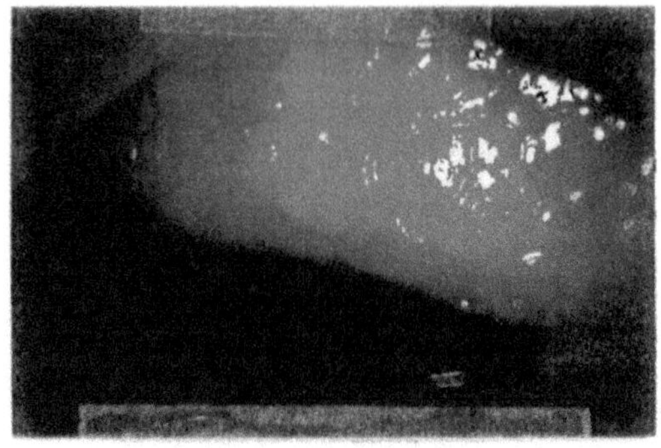

8

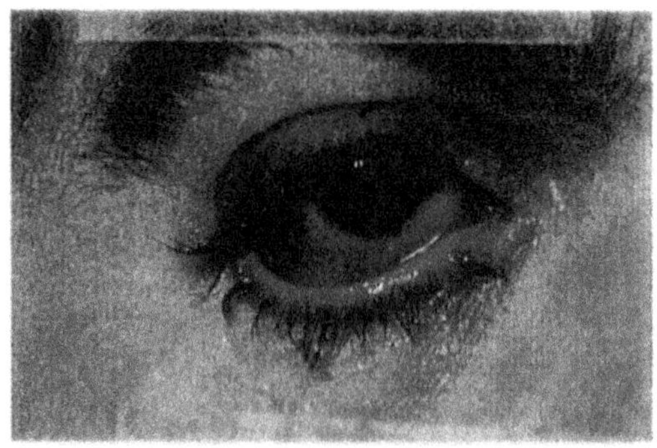

9

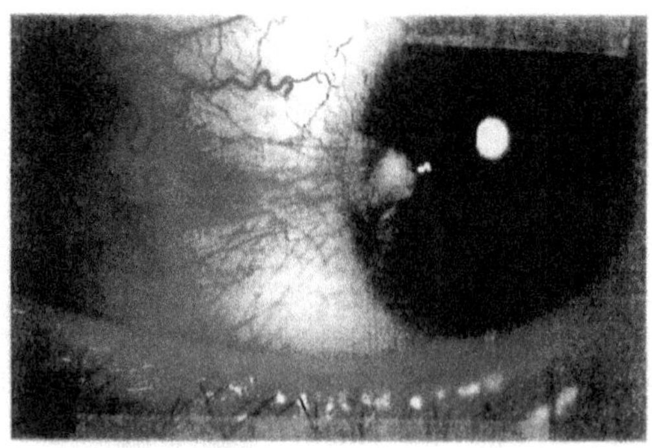

10

EXAMINATION SECTION

TEST 1

DIRECTIONS: Use the patient information provided to answer the questions that follow. Each question or incomplete statement is followed by several suggested answers or completions. Select the one that BEST answers the question or completes the statement. *PRINT THE LETTER OF THE CORRECT ANSWER IN THE SPACE AT THE RIGHT.*

Demographics: 40-year-old male
Chief complaint: Inability to close right eye completely – one month
Secondary complaints/symptoms: Diminution of vision in right eye – 15 days; dryness in right eye – 15 days
Patient's ocular history: nil
Patient's medical history: nil
Medications taken by patient: Topical ciprofloxacin drops
Patient's allergy history: nil
Family ocular history: nil
Family medical history: nil
Clinical findings: BCVA – OD-6/12; OS-6/6
Pupils: NSNR B/E
Confrontation fields: Full in both eyes
Slit lamp: Superficial punctate keratopathy in right eye, rest anterior and posterior segment in both eyes are normal
IOP: OD=OS=18 mmHg by applanation tonometry
Fundus: Both eyes – within normal limits

1. What is the most likely diagnosis of this condition? 1.______
   A. Exposure keratopathy
   B. Viral keratitis
   C. Common canalicular block
   D. Conjunctival xerosis

2. What can be the cause of this condition in this patient? 2.______
   A. Lacrimal gland carcinoma
   B. Bell's palsy
   C. Burns
   D. Chemical injury

3. All of the following can cause this condition EXCEPT 3.______
   A. severe proptosis
   B. cicatricial lid disease
   C. during sleep in some persons
   D. iron deficiency

4. Tests which are helpful in diagnosing exposure keratopathy include all of the following EXCEPT 4.______
   A. Schirmer's test
   B. tear film break up time
   C. Jone's dye test
   D. slit lamp exam for SPK

5. The neurological causes of exposure keratopathy include all EXCEPT 5.______
   A. idiopathic seventh nerve palsy
   B. diabetes mellitus
   C. acoustic neuroma
   D. fifth nerve palsy

Demographics: 40-year-old male
Chief complaint: Redness in one quadrant of right eye which is touching the cornea and extending 5 mm from it toward the fornix
Secondary complaints/symptoms: Mild ocular irritation, watering, photophobia in right eye
Patient's ocular history: Similar lesion appeared in right cornea one year ago, which was cured with patching and use of lubricants
Patient's medical history: no systemic disease
Medications taken by patient: Topical artificial tears
Patient's allergy history: nil
Family ocular history: nil
Family medical history: Father had diabetes
Clinical findings: BCVA – OD-6/9; OS-6/6
Pupils: NSNR B/E
Confrontation fields: Full in both eyes
Slit lamp: Fluorescein staining at periphery of cornea near the area of conjunctival and ciliary congestion
IOP: OD=OS=16 mmHg by applanation tonometry
Fundus: Both eyes – within normal limits

6. What is the most likely diagnosis of this condition? 6.______
   A. Peripheral corneal ulcer
   B. Diabetes mellitus related keratitis
   C. Superficial punctate keratitis
   D. Herpetic keratitis

7. What are the possible causes of this condition? 7.______
   A. Phylectenulosis
   B. Mooren's ulcer
   C. Dellen
   D. All of the above

8. The characteristic clinical features of Rosacea keratitis include all of the following EXCEPT 8.______
   A. it is more common in males
   B. hyperemia of face involving nose, central forehead and upper cheeks
   C. can cause corneal perforation
   D. can cause corneal neovascularisation

9. The features of Terrien's marginal degeneration include 9.______
   A. it is usually bilateral
   B. astigmatism
   C. pseudopterygium formation
   D. all of the above

10. The systemic diseases which can cause peripheral corneal thinning include all of the following EXCEPT 10.______
    A. rheumatoid arthritis
    B. polyarteritis nodosa
    C. systemic lupus erythematosus
    D. iron deficiency anemia

Demographics: 20-year-old male
Chief complaint: Excessive irritation in right eye from using RGP contact lenses for one month though he had been using these for last one year. Rapid relief when the lens is removed.
Secondary complaints/symptoms: Redness in right eye
Patient's ocular history: Myopia of –3 D in both eyes
Patient's medical history: nil
Medications taken by patient: Topical preservative-free artificial tears
Patient's allergy history: nil
Family ocular history: nil
Family medical history: nil
Clinical findings: BCVA (with contact lenses) – OD=OS=6/6
Pupils: NSNR in B/E
Confrontation fields: Full in B/E
Slit lamp: The rigid contact lens edge is chipped
IOP: 20 mmHg OS=OD by applanation tonometry
Fundus: Within normal limits

11. The RGP lens fit is not assessed by 11.______
    A. lens position and movement
    B. size of palpebral aperture following contact lens insertion
    C. fluorescein pattern
    D. comfort

12. A good fit of the RGP lens is shown by 12.______
    A. apical central clearance with light fluorescein centrally, absence of fluorescein in mid-peripheral area and band of fluorescein under periphery
    B. pooling of fluorescein centrally and absence of fluorescein under peripheral curves
    C. absence of fluorescein centrally and pooling of fluorescein under edges
    D. all of the above

13. Which of the following steps is not used to correct the fit of the contact lens? 13.______
    A. To tighten the fit, steepen the base curve or increase the diameter
    B. To loosen the fit, flatten the base curve or reduce the diameter
    C. Return the lens to laboratory for reblending
    D. Tint the contact lens

14. The clinical features which call for immediate discontinuation of RGP lenses are 14.______
    A. visual changes
    B. blurring of vision after lens removal
    C. excessive irritation
    D. all of the above

15. This patient's excessive irritation from wearing RGP lenses might NOT be due to 15.______
    A. solution sensitivity B. dry eyes
    C. angle closure glaucoma D. tear film problems

16. The principles followed for fitting RGP lenses include 16.______
    A. fit the smallest lens B. fit the thinnest lens
    C. should be no apical touch D. all of the above

Demographics: 50-year-old male
Chief complaint: Mild pain, redness and diminution of vision in both eyes
Secondary complaints/symptoms: Heaviness of both eyes
Patient's ocular history: nil
Patient's medical history: Patient is known diabetic for two years
Medications taken by patient: Anti-diabetics only; no ocular medications
Patient's allergy history: nil
Family ocular history: Father had open angle glaucoma
Family medical history: nil
Clinical findings: BCVA – R/E-6/9; L/E-6/9
Pupils: NSNR B/E
Humphery's Field analyzer: Enlargement of blind spot in both eyes
Slit lamp: Anterior segment is normal; gonioscopy shows open anterior chamber angle in both eyes
IOP: 28 mmHg in both eyes
Fundus: C:D:: 0.5:1 in both eyes, Laminar dot sign positive in both eyes

17. Which of the following statements is incorrect? 17.______
    A. Mackay Marg tonometer can be used on scarred or regular corneas
    B. Perkins tonometer needs a slit lamp to measure IOP
    C. With "air-puff" tonometer, there is no danger of spreading infection from one patient to another
    D. The Goldman tonometer is a variable force applanation tonometer

18. The C-value below which of the following is considered pathological? 18.______
    A. 0.11 B. 0.20 C. 0.19 D. 0.15

19. The anterior chamber angle can not be visualized with usual torch light examination because 19.______
    A. sclera at limbus covers the anterior chamber angle
    B. anterior chamber angle is transparent
    C. light emitted from angle structure undergoes total internal reflection
    D. all of the above

20. Which is a direct goniolens providing a mirror image of the same side angle? 20.______
    A. Goldman goniolens
    B. Zeiss goniolens
    C. Koeppe's goniolens
    D. None of the above

21. During the study of angle structures with gonioscopy, the most anterior structure is 21.______
    A. Schwalbe's line
    B. trabeculum
    C. Schlemm's canal
    D. scleral spur

22. Which of the following is incorrect regarding Grade 4 anterior chamber angle? 22.______
    A. Found in phakic patients
    B. Found in high myopia
    C. Ciliary body can be visualized
    D. Not capable of closure

23. The anterior chamber angle is most narrow when 23.______
    A. iris insertion is above Schwalbe's line
    B. iris insertion is behind Schwalbe's line
    C. iris root is at level of the scleral spur
    D. iris root is behind the scleral spur

24. Which of the following is false? 24.______
    A. The optic cup is a channel through which retinal nerve fibers leave the globe
    B. The optic cup represents volume of the channel not occupied by neural disc tissue
    C. The optic cup is bigger in larger optic discs
    D. The pathological cupping is caused by a decrease in the number of nerve fibers

25. What is the least suspicious factor of a glaucomatous cup among those given below? 25.______
    A. Asymmetrical cups in both eyes
    B. Larger cup in both eyes
    C. The cup size is found to be increasing
    D. The size of cupping and pallor both are increasing simultaneously

26. Which of these is not a glaucomatous field defect? 26.______
    A. Paracentral scotoma
    B. Nasal step
    C. Arcuate Bjerrum scotoma
    D. Temporal peripheral island

KEY (CORRECT ANSWERS)

1. A	11. B	21. A
2. B	12. A	22. A
3. D	13. D	23. A
4. C	14. D	24. A
5. D	15. C	25. B
6. A	16. D	26. D
7. D	17. B	
8. A	18. A	
9. D	19. C	
10. D	20. C	

TEST 2

DIRECTIONS: Use the patient information provided to answer the questions that follow. Each question or incomplete statement is followed by several suggested answers or completions. Select the one that BEST answers the question or completes the statement. *PRINT THE LETTER OF THE CORRECT ANSWER IN THE SPACE AT THE RIGHT.*

Demographics: 15-year-old female
Chief complaint: Discomfort while wearing soft contact lenses with increasing lens awareness in both eyes
Secondary complaints/symptoms: Redness of eyes, foreign body sensation, itching and mucoid discharge in both eyes
Patient's ocular history: Patient had –4 D of myopia
Patient's medical history: nil
Medications taken by patient: nil
Patient's allergy history: nil
Family ocular history: Mother had myopia
Family medical history: nil
Clinical findings: BCVA – 6/5 in both eyes
Pupils: NSNR in both eyes
Confrontation fields: Full in both eyes
Slit lamp: The slit lamp examination does not show a normal contact lens mobility during blinking. On averting the upper eyelids, papillary hyperplasia is visible. Papillae measure 0.3 mm to 1 mm.
IOP: OD=OS=17 mmHg by applanation tonometry
Fundus: Both eyes – within normal limits

1. What is the most likely cause of this condition? 1.______
   A. Allergic conjunctivitis B. Corneal edema
   C. Giant papillary conjunctivitis D. All of the above

2. What is the chemical in contact lens solution that can cause both allergic conjunctivitis and giant papillary conjunctivitis? 2.______
   A. Thiomersal B. Hydrogen peroxide
   C. Topical antibiotic solution D. Topical steroids

3. The corneal complications of soft contact lenses include 3.______
   A. epithelial edema B. abrasions
   C. corneal infiltrates D. all of the above

4. Which is NOT the basic lens parameter of primary importance for fitting contact lenses? 4.______
   A. Base curve B. Power
   C. Diameter D. Condition of optic nerve

5. The disadvantages of soft contact lenses as compared to RGP lenses do NOT include 5.______
   A. lower quality of vision B. more deposits
   C. lower cost D. uncorrected astigmatism

6. The test that can evaluate whether soft contact lenses fit properly include all of the following EXCEPT 6.______
   A. movement with blink B. retinoscopy
   C. keratometry D. ophthalmoscopy

7. The signs of chronic hypoxia from contact lens wear does NOT include 7.______
   A. punctate staining B. epithelial microcysts
   C. stromal edema D. iritis

Demographics: 40-year-old male
Chief complaint: A red nodule on sclera in right eye
Secondary complaints/symptoms: Mild discomfort, tenderness to touch, watering
Patient's ocular history: Similar history of appearance of nodule in the past
Patient's medical history: nil
Medications taken by patient: Topical corticosteroids
Patient's allergy history: nil
Family ocular history: nil
Family medical history: nil
Clinical findings: BCVA – 6/6 in both eyes
Pupils: B/E NSNR
Confrontation fields: Normal
Slit lamp: Nodules on sclera with congestion of episcleral vessels
IOP: 18 mmHg OS=OD by applanation tonometry
Fundus: Within normal limits

8. What is the most likely diagnosis of this condition? 8.______
   A. Episcleritis B. Pterygium
   C. Pingecula D. Trabecular bleb

9. Which of the following statements is NOT correct? 9.______
   A. Episcleritis is seldom associated with systemic disease
   B. Scleritis is seldom associated with systemic disease
   C. Pain is more in scleritis than episcleritis
   D. Scleritis can be caused by herpes zoster

10. Systemic anti-inflammatory agents and immunosuppresants are needed for treatment of 10.______
   A. scleritis B. episcleritis
   C. phylectenular conjunctivitis D. all of the above

11. The following are all various types of scleritis EXCEPT 11.______
    A. posterior scleritis
    B. acute necrotizing scleritis with inflammation
    C. acute necrotizing scleritis without inflammation
    D. equatorial scleritis

12. Which of the following is a complication of scleritis? 12.______
    A. Thinned sclera
    B. Secondary glaucoma
    C. Exudative retinal detachment
    D. All of the above

Demographics: 15-year-old male
Chief complaint: Recurrent redness of left eye and diminution of vision in left eye for two years
Secondary complaints/symptoms: Mild irritation, photophobia, pain, lacrimation in left eye
Patient's ocular history: Vesicular eruptions on tip of nose extending on to the forehead on left side of face with involvement of cornea two years ago
Patient's medical history: nil
Medications taken by patient: Topical corticosteroids for present complaint
Patient's allergy history: nil
Family ocular history: Not significant
Family medical history: nil
Clinical findings: BCVA – R/E 6/6, L/E 6/24
Pupils: R/E – NSNR; L/E – constricted with posterior synechiae
Confrontation fields: R/E – normal; L/E – decreased
Slit lamp: R/E – normal; L/E – circumcorneal congestion, powdery keratic precipitates on back of cornea, aqueous flare-positive, posterior synechiae-positive
IOP: R/E – 16 mmHg; L/E – 20 mmHg
Fundus: Central fundus in both eyes is normal

13. What is the most likely diagnosis of this condition? 13.______
    A. Herpes zoster associated with anterior uveitis
    B. Granulomatous uveitis
    C. Choroiditis
    D. Optic neuritis

14. What can be the coexistent clinical features of herpes zoster anterior uveitis? 14.______
    A. Decrease in corneal sensitivity
    B. Nummular lesions in corneal stroma
    C. Patches of iris atrophy
    D. All of the above

15. The diseases which essentially have powdery keratic precipitates are all of the following EXCEPT 15.______
    A. herpes zoster
    B. ankylosing spondylitis
    C. Behcet's disease
    D. leprosy

16. The pathogenesis of iridocyclitis in herpes simplex can be 16.______
    A. exogenous
    B. endogenous
    C. both A and B
    D. none of the above

17. The non-infectious systemic diseases that can cause iridocyclitis include all of the following EXCEPT 17.______
    A. sarcoidosis
    B. Behcet's disease
    C. Vogt Koyanagi disease
    D. syphilis

18. Uveitis is usually bilateral in all EXCEPT 18.______
    A. syphilis
    B. tuberculosis
    C. ankylosing spondylitis
    D. leprosy

19. Immunosuppresants should be avoided in uveitis due to 19.______
    A. Behcet's disease
    B. sarcoidosis
    C. sympathetic ophthalmitis
    D. herpes simplex

20. Acute retinal necrosis can be caused by 20.______
    A. cytomegalovirus
    B. herpes zoster ophthalmicus
    C. both A and B
    D. none of the above

21. Which is not true about presumed ocular histoplasmosis syndrome? 21.______
    A. The fungus Histoplasma capsulatum has been recovered from an eye with presumed ocular histoplasmosis syndrome
    B. The disease has an increased prevalence in areas where histoplasmosis is endemic
    C. Histoplasmin skin test is positive in 90% of patients with POHS
    D. Subretinal neovascular membrane may be present at macula

22. Which of the following applies to sympathetic ophthalmitis? 22.______
    A. Panuveitis
    B. Bilateral
    C. Granulomatous
    D. All of the above

23. The earliest feature of inflammation in sympathesizing eye is 23.______
    A. Koeppe nodules
    B. cells in retrolental space
    C. mutton fat keratic precipitates
    D. iris thickening

24. To prevent sympathetic ophthalmitis, within two weeks of injury the exciting eye should be 24.______
    A. enucleated B. eviscerated
    C. both A and B D. neither A nor B

25. Which is NOT true about acute retinal necrosis? 25.______
    A. It is bilateral in 30-50% of cases
    B. In cases with involvement of peripheral fundus, the visual acuity remains fairly good
    C. It resolves within 4-12 weeks
    D. Exudative retinal detachment is common

26. The "three C's" of congenital toxoplasmosis do NOT include 26.______
    A. convulsions B. chorioretinitis
    C. corneal edema D. calcification

27. The drug most commonly used for treatment of ocular toxoplasmosis is 27.______
    A. clindamycin B. sulphonamide
    C. pyrimethamine D. all of the above

28. The main complication of anterior uveitis due to herpes zoster virus can be 28.______
    A. oculomotor nerve palsy B. proptosis
    C. iris atrophy D. none of the above

29. The organisms which cause opportunistic infection in patients with AIDS are 29.______
    A. Ebstein Barr virus B. herpes zoster
    C. pneumocystis carnii D. all of the above

30. Cystoid macular edema is found in 30.______
    A. pars planitis B. Behcet's disease
    C. sarcoidosis D. all of the above

KEY (CORRECT ANSWERS)

1. C	11. D	21. A
2. A	12. D	22. D
3. D	13. A	23. B
4. D	14. D	24. A
5. C	15. D	25. D
6. D	16. C	26. C
7. D	17. D	27. D
8. A	18. C	28. C
9. B	19. D	29. D
10. A	20. C	30. D

EXAMINATION SECTION

TEST 1

DIRECTIONS: Use the patient information provided to answer the questions that follow. Each question or incomplete statement is followed by several suggested answers or completions. Select the one that BEST answers the question or completes the statement. *PRINT THE LETTER OF THE CORRECT ANSWER IN THE SPACE AT THE RIGHT.*

Demographics: 50-year-old female
Chief complaint: Mild heaviness and pain in both eyes – one month
Secondary complaints/symptoms: nil
Patient's ocular history: Itching, redness, watering in both eyes (two months), for which she used topical steroids, four times a day for one month
Patient's medical history: nil
Medications taken by patient: Topical corticosteroids, four times a day for one month
Patient's allergy history: Allergic rhinitis
Family ocular history: nil
Family medical history: nil
Clinical findings: BCVA – OD=OS-6/6
Pupils: NSNR B/E
Confrontation fields: Full in both eyes
Slit lamp: Both upper lids show papillary hyperplasia, anterior segment is normal, anterior chamber was open in both eyes
IOP: OD=OS=26 mmHg by applanation tonometry
Fundus: C:D::0.4:1 in both eyes; foveal reflex – normal in both eyes

1. What is the most likely diagnosis of this patient? 1.______
   A. Primary open angle glaucoma
   B. Primary angle closure glaucoma
   C. High corticosteroid responder
   D. Trachoma

2. Which of the following statements is correct? 2.______
   A. 40% of patients with established POAG are high corticosteroid reactors
   B. The response of IOP to topical corticosteroid administration is determined genetically
   C. Both high myopes and diabetics have a higher incidence of corticosteroid responsiveness
   D. All of the above

3. Which of the following statements is NOT correct? 3.______
   A. Topical corticosteroid should be used with caution in patients with POAG and in their first degree relative
   B. Systemic corticosteroid cause elevation of IOP as much as topical preparations
   C. Fluoromethalone raises the IOP half as much as betamethasone
   D. Clobetasone has a low propensity for elevating IOP

4. The ocular association of POAG does NOT include 4.______
   A. high myopia
   B. retinal vein occlusion
   C. exudative retinal detachment
   D. retinitis pigmentosa

5. The systemic association of POAG does NOT include 5.______
   A. diabetes mellitus
   B. phenylthiocarbamide tasting
   C. low levels of protein bound iodine
   D. hyperparathyroidism

Demographics: 45-year-old female
Chief complaint: Mild pain and redness in both eyes for one year
Secondary complaints/symptoms: nil
Patient's ocular history: nil
Patient's medical history: nil
Medications taken by patient: nil
Patient's allergy history: nil
Family ocular history: Mother turned blind in one eye after having similar history
Family medical history: nil
Clinical findings: BCVA – OS=OD=6/9
Pupils: NSNR in both eyes
Confrontation fields: Normal in both eyes
Slit lamp: Anterior chamber is about 1 mm deep in both eyes; there is a narrow entrance to the chamber angle
IOP: 26 mmHg in both eyes
Fundus: C:D::0.5:1 in both eyes; foveal reflex – normal in both eyes

6. What is the likely diagnosis of this condition? 6.______
   A. Latent angle closure glaucoma
   B. Chronic angle closure glaucoma
   C. Acute angle closure glaucoma
   D. Intermittent angle closure glaucoma

7. Which clinical feature is NOT true for this condition? 7.______
   A. Angle becomes closed slowly and progressively
   B. Closure usually starts inferiorly and spreads superiorly
   C. The symptoms are same as the of POAG
   D. Cupping of optic disc and visual field loss is identical to that seen in POAG

8. Which is not true of indentation gonioscopy? 8.______
   A. It opens only appositional closure of angle and is not effective for opening the angle if it has synechial closure
   B. It forces aqueous into peripheral part of anterior chamber
   C. It forces peripheral iris away from angle structures
   D. It can tear away adhesions from trabeculum if synechial closure of angle is present

9. Which is true about latent angle closure glaucoma? 9.______
   A. The eye with latent angle closure glaucoma has raised IOP
   B. Peripheral iridectomy is not advised in eyes with latent phase angle closure glaucoma if the fellow eye has suffered an acute or subacute attack of PACG
   C. Provocative tests are useful to determine if angle is capable of closure
   D. All of the above

10. What is not true of the provocative tests in angle closure glaucoma? 10.______
    A. Dark room test is a provocative test
    B. Prone-Dark room test is a physiological provocative test
    C. In a pharmacological provocative test, 10% phenylephrine combined with 2% pilocarpine is used
    D. None of the above

11. The mydriatic provocative tests 11.______
    A. are unphysiological
    B. may precipitate a severe attack of angle closure glaucoma
    C. can cause elevation of IOP even in the presence of an open angle
    D. are all of the above

Demographics: 40-year-old male
Chief complaint: Severe pain, redness, watering and diminution of vision in right eye for one month
Secondary complaints/symptoms: Photophobia in right eye
Patient's ocular history: Recurrent redness of right eye for two years
Patient's medical history: Not significant
Medications taken by patient: Frequent topical steroids for above complaints
Patient's allergy history: nil
Family ocular history: nil
Family medical history: nil
Clinical findings: BCVA – R/E: 6/36; L/E: 6/6
Pupils: R/E – pupil constricted and not reacting to light; L/E – normal
Confrontation fields: R/E – constricted; L/E – normal
Slit lamp: R/E – pigmented keratic precipitates, occlusio pupillae, iris bombe, aqueous flare; L/E – normal
IOP: R/E – 28 mmHg; L/E – 18 mmHg
Fundus: R/E – C:D::0.5:1, foveal reflex is normal; L/E – C:D::0.3:1, foveal reflex is normal

12. What is the most likely diagnosis of this condition? 12.______
    A. Primary angle closure glaucoma
    B. Secondary angle closure glaucoma
    C. Primary open angle glaucoma
    D. None of the above

13. Formation of peripheral anterior synechiae causing angle closure is more common 13.______
    A. in eyes with granulomatous inflammation
    B. in eyes with non-granulomatous inflammation
    C. when incidence is equal in both eyes
    D. none of the above

14. Continuous serial monitoring of IOP is needed in such patients as 14.______
    A. IOP may fluctuate depending on the ciliary body status
    B. even severe elevations of IOP up to 50 mmHg may be asymptomatic as previous rise in IOP had been slow
    C. even glaucomatous eyes with IOP of 35 mmHg may become hypotonous during acute exacerbations
    D. all of the above

15. Neovascular glaucoma is not found in which of the following conditions? 15.______
    A. Diabetes mellitus
    B. Central retinal vein occlusion
    C. Central choroiditis
    D. Eales' disease

16. The open anterior chamber angle along with raised IOP can be found in patients of iridocyclitis in all of these conditions EXCEPT 16.______
    A. trabecular obstruction due to inflammatory cells and debris
    B. acute trabeculitis
    C. steroid induced
    D. trabecular obstruction due to PAS

5 (#1)

Demographics: 60-year-old male
Chief complaint: Diminution of vision in right eye for two months, and in left eye for three months
Secondary complaints/symptoms: Mild dryness of both eyes
Patient's ocular history: nil
Patient's medical history: Patient is diabetic
Medications taken by patient: Antidiabetic medications
Patient's allergy history: nil
Family ocular history: Both mother and father were operated on for cataracts in both eyes
Family medical history: History of diabetes is positive
Clinical findings: BCVA – OD=OS=6/36
Pupils: NSNR in both eyes
Confrontation fields: OD=OS=normal
Slit lamp: Immature senile cataract in both eyes, rest anterior segment within normal limits
IOP: 20 mmHg in both eyes
Fundus: On fluoroscein angiography, hemorrhages and exudates in both eyes, dull foveal reflex in both eyes

17. Which examination technique on this patient would be most appropriate for determining both diagnosis and prognosis? 17.______
    A. Fluoroscein angiography
    B. Tonography
    C. Laser inferometry
    D. Indirect ophthalmoscopy

18. Which are the vessels that allow leakage of free fluoroscein into extravascular space in a healthy subject? 18.______
    A. Retinal capillary endothelium
    B. Major choroidal vessels
    C. Choriocapillaries
    D. Across retinal pigment epithelium

19. The C value in tonography of a normal individual is ______ μl/min/mmHg. 19.______
    A. 0.28
    B. 0.18
    C. 0.13
    D. None of the above

20. Which of the following statements is correct regarding indirect ophthalmoscopy? 20.______
    A. 30 D lens has 60° field of view and twice the magnification
    B. 20 D lens has 30° field of view and four times the magnification
    C. 14 D lens has 51° field of view and thrice the magnification
    D. All of the above

21. In fluoroscein angiography, which of the following statements is correct? 21.______
   A. Blue light enters the eye due to blue excitation filters
   B. Yellow-green light enters the camera due to use of yellow-green barrier filter
   C. White light is emitted from retinal camera
   D. All of the above

22. Hypofluorescence in fluoroscein angiography cannot be due to 22.______
   A. blockage of fluorescence due to increased density of xanthophylls in neurosensory retina
   B. leakage of dye from choroidal or retinal neovascularisation
   C. blockage of fluorescence due to increased density of melanin in retinal pigment epithelium
   D. obstruction of retinal or choroidal circulation

23. Which if the following is NOT associated with subretinal neovascular membrane? 23.______
   A. Choroidal rupture B. Best's disease
   C. Rubella retinopathy D. Severe hypermetropia

24. Which of the following show fluoroscein staining? 24.______
   I. Optic disc
   II. Sclera
   III. Drusen
   IV. Fibrous scar tissue

   A. Only I B. I and II C. I, II and III D. All of them

25. Hyperfluorescence in fluoroscein angiography cannot be due to 25.______
   A. increased quantity of extravascular fluoroscein leakage into serous or hemorrhagic areas
   B. drusens
   C. decrease in the filter effect of pigment epithelium
   D. vascular tumors

KEY (CORRECT ANSWERS)

1. C	11. D	21. D
2. D	12. B	22. B
3. B	13. A	23. D
4. C	14. D	24. D
5. D	15. C	25. D
6. B	16. D	
7. B	17. A	
8. D	18. C	
9. C	19. A	
10. D	20. A	

TEST 2

DIRECTIONS: Use the patient information provided to answer the questions that follow. Each question or incomplete statement is followed by several suggested answers or completions. Select the one that BEST answers the question or completes the statement. *PRINT THE LETTER OF THE CORRECT ANSWER IN THE SPACE AT THE RIGHT.*

Demographics: 50-year-old male
Chief complaint: Heaviness and pain in both eyes – one year
Secondary complaints/symptoms: nil
Patient's ocular history: nil
Patient's medical history: nil
Medications taken by patient: nil
Patient's allergy history: nil
Family ocular history: Father had POAG
Family medical history: Father had diabetes
Clinical findings: BCVA – OD=OS=6/5
Pupils: NSNR B/E
Central 30° Fields: Paracentral scotoma in both eyes
Slit lamp: Anterior segment normal, open anterior chamber angles
IOP: 20 mmHg in both eyes
Fundus: C:D::0.5:1 in both eyes; foveal reflex – normal in both eyes

1. What is the likely diagnosis of this condition? 1.______
   A. POAG
   B. PACG
   C. Low tension glaucoma
   D. None of the above

2. Which of the following cannot lead to the condition mentioned above? 2.______
   A. Sudden profound systemic hypotension
   B. Acute blood loss
   C. Myocardial infarction
   D. Vasovagal syncope

3. The mimicking condition of this disease is 3.______
   A. congenital optic disc anomalies
   B. colobomatous optic disc
   C. compressive or ischemic optic nerve or chiasmal lesion
   D. all of the above

4. The drug of choice for treatment of this condition is 4.______
   A. brimonidine or latanoprost
   B. timolol or brimonidine
   C. timolol or latanoprost
   D. none of the above

5. Which is a technique used to measure ocular blood flow? 5.______
   A. Colour Doppler ultrasonography
   B. Scanning laser Doppler flowmetry
   C. Pulsatile ocular blood flow tonometer
   D. All of the above

6. According to Normal Tension Glaucoma Study guidelines, the IOP should be lowered by ______ of the baseline. 6.______
   A. 30% B. 20%
   C. 10% D. Any of the above

7. The neuroprotectors include all of the following EXCEPT 7.______
   A. brimonidine B. free radical scavengers
   C. nitric oxide inhibitors D. timolol

Demographics: 2-year-old male
Chief complaint: Parents complain that they have seen white reflex in pupillary area of the child's right eye
Secondary complaints/symptoms: nil
Patient's ocular history: nil
Patient's medical history: nil
Medications taken by patient: nil
Patient's allergy history: nil
Family ocular history: Not significant
Family medical history: nil
Clinical findings: BCVA – not possible to record
Pupils: NSNR B/E
Confrontation Fields: Not possible to assess
Slit lamp: No other abnormality except white reflex in the pupil of right eye
IOP: 16 mmHg by applanation tonometry in both eyes
Fundus: In right eye it is not possible to see; in left eye, C:D::0.3:1, foveal reflex is normal

8. What is the most likely diagnosis of this condition? 8.______
   A. Congenital glaucoma
   B. Congenital cataract
   C. Congenital corneal opacity
   D. All of the above

9. Which of the following tests would not be appropriate for determining rubella? 9.______
   A. Serology typing for IgM rubella antibody
   B. Virus culture from the nasopharynx
   C. Platelet count for thrombocytopenia
   D. Urinalysis for reducing substances

10. Which of the following tests would determine the diagnosis of Lowe's syndrome? 10.______
    A. Serum calcium and phosphorus
    B. Urine chromatography for amino acids
    C. Blood glucose determination
    D. Red blood cells for galactokinase activity

11. Which test would be used to assess the visual function in the right eye of this patient? 11.______
    A. Visually evoked response
    B. Preferential looking
    C. Presence or absence of nystagmus and strabismus
    D. All of the above

12. Which disease is not associated with the above condition? 12.______
    A. Rubella
    B. Herpes zoster
    C. Galactosemia
    D. Hypocalcaemia

13. Which of the following is also a differential diagnosis of this condition? 13.______
    A. Persistent primary hyperplastic vitreous
    B. Retinoblastoma
    C. Coat's disease
    D. All of the above

Demographics: 50-year-old male
Chief complaint: Sudden painless diminution of vision upon rising from bed in morning
Secondary complaints/symptoms: nil
Patient's ocular history: nil
Patient's medical history: Patient is hypertensive with blood pressure in range of 150/90 mmHg. Patient also had fracture of the femur one month ago.
Medications taken by patient: nil
Patient's allergy history: nil
Family ocular history: Father was also hypertensive
Family medical history: nil
Clinical findings: BCVA – OS=OD=6/9
Pupils: NSNR
Confrontation Fields: Normal
Slit lamp: Anterior segment is normal in both eyes
IOP: 20 mmHg in both eyes
Fundus: Arterio-venous crossing changes in both eyes

14. What is the most likely diagnosis of this condition? 14.______
    A. Central retinal vein occlusion
    B. Vitreous hemorrhage
    C. Central retinal artery occlusion
    D. Thrombocytopenia

15. What is the probable systemic cause related to the ocular disease in this patient? 15.______
    A. Hypertension
    B. Fractured femur
    C. Both A and B
    D. There is no relation to systemic factors

16. What cannot be a complication of this ocular condition? 16.______
    A. Cystoid macular edema
    B. Glaucoma
    C. Vitreous hemorrhage
    D. Retinal detachment

17. What is the name given to the retinopathy caused in this condition? 17.______
    A. Blood and thunder retinopathy
    B. Eale's disease
    C. Coat's disease
    D. Retinopathy of prematurity

18. What is not found in fundus of a patient with this ocular disease? 18.______
    A. Dot and blot hemorrhages
    B. Flame-shaped hemorrhage
    C. Bone spicule pigmentation
    D. Cotton wool spots

19. In this condition, what is the clinical feature that cannot differentiate acute from chronic stage? 19.______
    A. Venous sheathing
    B. Chronic cystoid macular edema
    C. Collateral formation
    D. Central retinal artery occlusion

Demographics: 55-year-old female
Chief complaint: Diminution of vision in left eye. She wants to know visual results she should expect following cataract surgery in left eye.
Secondary complaints/symptoms: nil
Patient's ocular history: Cataract surgery in right eye one year ago in which she did not gain useful vision, and the only vision possible was 6/36.
Patient's medical history: nil
Medications taken by patient: nil
Patient's allergy history: nil
Family ocular history: Not significant
Family medical history: nil
Clinical findings: BCVA – OD < 6/60; OS = 6/36
Pupils: NSNR in both eyes
Confrontation Fields: Not possible in right eye due to opaque media; in left eye fields appear normal
Slit lamp: Within normal limits
IOP: 18 mmHg in both eyes
Fundus: OD – not visible; OS – C:D::0.3:1; subretinal neovascular membrane at macula

20. Which test can you advise to determine the visual results expected in the right eye following cataract surgery? 20.______
    A. Potential visual acuity meter
    B. Laser inferometry
    C. Focal ERG
    D. All of the above

21. Which statement is incorrect regarding laser inferometry? 21.______
    A. The alternate pattern of light and dark fringes is known as interference pattern
    B. If the waves are 180° out of place, maxima adds to the minima and a destructive interference occurs
    C. A pair of coherent light sources – a split He- Ne laser beam is used to form interference pattern
    D. If waves are in phase with each other, the maxima adds to minima resulting in a wave which is eight times the intensity of the initial wave

22. Potential acuity meter is useful in determining post operative visual acuity in patients with 22.______
    A. dense cataract
    B. immature senile cataract
    C. macular holes
    D. macular edema

23. Pinhole does not lead to improvement in visual acuity in patients with 23.______
    A. refractive error
    B. peripheral corneal opacities
    C. central lenticular opacities
    D. peripheral lenticular opacities

24. In macular diseases, which does NOT hold true? 24.______
    A. Normal amplitude of Flash ERG
    B. Normal ratio of EOG
    C. Decreased amplitude of Pattern ERG
    D. Decreased amplitude of Flash ERG

25. In optic nerve diseases, which statement is correct? 25.______
    A. Flash ERG has decreased amplitude
    B. EOG has reduced ratio
    C. VEP has increased latency
    D. None of the above

KEY (CORRECT ANSWERS)

1. C	11. D	21. D
2. D	12. B	22. B
3. D	13. D	23. C
4. A	14. A	24. D
5. D	15. A	25. C
6. A	16. D	
7. D	17. A	
8. B	18. C	
9. D	19. D	
10. B	20. D	

EXAMINATION SECTION

TEST 1

DIRECTIONS: Use the patient information provided to answer the questions that follow. Each question or incomplete statement is followed by several suggested answers or completions. Select the one that BEST answers the question or completes the statement. *PRINT THE LETTER OF THE CORRECT ANSWER IN THE SPACE AT THE RIGHT.*

Demographics: 65-year-old male
Chief complaint: Painless, progressive diminution of vision for two years
Secondary complaints/symptoms: nil
Patient's ocular history: Had cataract surgery in both eyes with IOL implantation followed by gain of useful vision
Patient's medical history: Not significant
Medications taken by patient: Nil
Patient's allergy history: Nil
Family ocular history: Not significant
Family medical history: Not significant
Clinical findings: BCVA – OD 6/12, OS 6/24
Pupils: NSNR
Confrontation fields: Appear to be normal in both eyes
Slit lamp: Anterior segment appears normal
IOP: 18 mmHg in both eyes
Fundus: Soft drusen in foveal region in both eyes

1. What can be the cause for the sudden loss of vision in this patient? 1.______
   A. Hemorrhagic detachment of retinal pigment epithelium
   B. Hemorrhagic detachment of neurosensory retina
   C. Vitreous hemorrhage
   D. All of the above

2. The manifestations of age-related macular degeneration on fluorescein angiography is 2.______
   A. early hyperfluorescence due to filling of vessels
   B. late hyperfluorescence due to staining of fibrous tissues
   C. SRNVM fluoresces
   D. all of the above

3. What is the role of fluorescein angiography if one needs to determine the prognosis of ARMD? 3.______
   I. size of lesion II. predominantly classic
   III. predominantly occult

   A. I and II B. II and III C. I and III D. I, II and III

4. How is ICG angiography better than fluorescein angiography for diagnosis of this condition? 4.______
   A. No masking of choroidal circulation by ocular pigment and blood
   B. Protein bound thus no leaking from choroidal circulation
   C. Both of the above
   D. None of the above

5. What are the conditions in which ICG is better than FA for diagnosis? 5.______
   A. ARMD
   B. Idiopathic polypoidal choroidal vascularisation
   C. Occult choroidal neovascular membrane
   D. All of the above

6. Drusens are focal collections of hyaline material between 6.______
   A. basal lamina of retinal pigment epithelium and the inner collagenous layer of Bruch's membrane
   B. outer pigment epithelium and inner pigment epithelium
   C. choroids and Bruch's membrane
   D. none of the above

7. The staining of drusens with fluorescein can be differentiated from leakage of dye because 7.______
   A. fluorescein is well defined
   B. actual dimensions of hyperfluorescent area seen 20 minutes after dye injection are the same as during the early stages of dye transit
   C. more prolonged time of fluorescence is seen in staining of drusen than in leakage
   D. all of the above

8. Which factors are associated with increased risk of visual loss? 8.______
   I. Focal hyperpigmentation
   II. Confluent drusens
   III. Exudative ARMD
   IV. One eye has already developed visual loss from ARMD

   A. I and II
   B. I, II, III and IV
   C. II, III and IV
   D. I and IV

9. Which of the following is not true regarding dry ARMD? 9.______
   A. Most common type of ARMD
   B. Causes rapid loss of vision
   C. Is due to slow and progressive atrophy of retinal pigment epithelium
   D. No effective treatment of visual loss except low vision aids

10. The monitoring of the visual function in ARMD includes all EXCEPT 10.______
    A. measurement both for near and distance visual acuity
    B. area of scotoma or visual distortion documented on Amsler's grid
    C. excimer laser therapy
    D. fluorescein angiography

Demographics: 30-year-old male
Chief complaint: Sudden loss of vision in right eye
Secondary complaints/symptoms: Blurring of vision in right eye; distortion of lines
Patient's ocular history: Similar complaint one year ago – resolved spontaneously
Patient's medical history: Nil
Medications taken by patient: Nil
Patient's allergy history: Nil
Family ocular history: Nil
Family medical history: Nil
Clinical findings: BCVA – OD 6/12 corrected to 6/6 with addition of weak 'plus' lenses; OS 6/6
Pupils: NSNR in both eyes
Confrontation fields: Fields normal in both eyes
Slit lamp: Anterior segment is normal
IOP: 16 mmHg in both eyes
Fundus: OD – C:D::0.3:1, foveal reflex is dull, I/O – a round elevation of sensory retina at the posterior pole; OS – C:D::0.3:1, foveal reflex is sharp

11. What is the most likely diagnosis of this condition? 11.______
    A. Retinal detachment
    B. Central serous retinopathy
    C. Confluent drusens
    D. Central retinal artery occlusion

12. Which diagnostic modality is the best one to make the diagnosis? 12.______
    A. Fluorescein angiography
    B. Indirect ophthalmoscopy
    C. Slit lamp examination with 90 D lens
    D. Direct ophthalmoscopy

13. Which ocular condition is most often associated with the above disease? 13.______
    A. Congenital optic disc pit
    B. Uveitis
    C. Age-related macular degeneration
    D. Diabetic retinopathy

14. What are the patterns seen in fluorescein angiography in this disease? 14.______
    I. Smokestack appearance
    II. Ink-blot appearance
    III. Flower petal pattern
    IV. Late staining in macular region

    A. I and II B. II and III C. III and IV D. I and IV

15. Which drugs have no role in treatment of the above disease? 15.______
    A. Antibiotics
    B. Steroids
    C. Analgesics
    D. Antifungals

16. The clinical features of the above disease including all of the following EXCEPT 16.______
    A. central scotoma
    B. ring reflex at macula in ophthalmoscopy
    C. blue colour dulled
    D. red colour dulled

17. The underlying pathology in this condition is 17.______
    A. malfunctioning of RPE pump
    B. atrophy of RPE
    C. hyperplasia of RPE
    D. all of the above

18. Which is true regarding the course of this disease? 18.______
    A. Heals spontaneously in 4-8 weeks
    B. All patients recover with laser treatment
    C. Laser treatment should be done as soon as diagnosis is made
    D. Steroids should be given systemically for symptomatic relief

19. Laser treatment is indicated 19.______
    A. in recurrent cases
    B. in bilateral cases
    C. for occupational reasons
    D. all of the above

20. Chronic idiopathic central serous chorioretinopathy can cause all of the following EXCEPT 20.______
    A. permanent loss of vision
    B. serous retinal detachment
    C. ARMD
    D. large RPE detachments

Demographics: 30-year-old male
Chief complaint: Sudden painless diminution of vision in right eye
Secondary complaints/symptoms: Nil
Patient's ocular history: Had complaint of vitreous floaters and blurring of vision in both eyes for one year (with right eye affected more than left eye)
Patient's medical history: Nil
Medications taken by patient: Systemic steroids previously
Patient's allergy history: Nil
Family ocular history: Nil
Family medical history: Father had pulmonary tuberculosis and was treated for nine months with antitubercular therapy
Clinical findings: BCVA – <6/60 in right eye; 6/18 in left eye
Pupils: NSNR in both eyes
Confrontation fields: Fields appear normal in both eyes
Slit lamp: Anterior segment is normal in both eyes
IOP: 18 mmHg in both eyes
Fundus: Right eye – no glow with reddish hue; Left eye – periphlebitis and some flame-shaped hemorrhages

21. What is the most likely diagnosis of this condition? 21.______
    A. Central retinal vein occlusion
    B. Diabetes retinopathy
    C. Eales' disease
    D. Central retinal artery occlusion

22. What are the known systemic associations with this disease? 22.______
    A. Tuberculosis
    B. Septic foci
    C. Allergies
    D. All of the above

23. Which statement is not true regarding Eales' disease? 23.______
    A. Macula is involved early
    B. Neovascularisation elsewhere is more common than neovascularisation disc
    C. Varying degree of peripheral retinal nonperfusion is seen
    D. Rapid occlusion of inflamed veins causes hemorrhages

24. The complications of Eales' disease do NOT include 24.______
    A. uveitis
    B. cataract
    C. rubeosis iridis
    D. corneal edema

25. The treatment modalities of Eales' disease include 25.______
    A. sarcoidosis
    B. uveitis
    C. syphilis
    D. all of the above

KEY (CORRECT ANSWERS)

1. D	11. B	21. C
2. D	12. A	22. D
3. D	13. A	23. A
4. C	14. A	24. D
5. D	15. B	25. D
6. A	16. C	
7. D	17. A	
8. B	18. A	
9. B	19. D	
10. C	20. C	

TEST 2

DIRECTIONS: Use the patient information provided to answer the questions that follow. Each question or incomplete statement is followed by several suggested answers or completions. Select the one that BEST answers the question or completes the statement. *PRINT THE LETTER OF THE CORRECT ANSWER IN THE SPACE AT THE RIGHT.*

Demographics: 50-year-old female
Chief complaint: Failure to gain expected vision following cataract extraction with IOL implantation in left eye
Secondary complaints/symptoms: nil
Patient's ocular history: nil
Patient's medical history: nil
Medications taken by patient: Nil
Patient's allergy history: Nil
Family ocular history: Nil
Family medical history: Nil
Clinical findings: BCVA – OD 6/12, OS 6/18
Pupils: NSNR in both eyes
Confrontation fields: Appear to be normal in both eyes
Slit lamp: Anterior segment is normal in both eyes, pulled up pupil in left eye
IOP: OD – 16mmHg; OS – 18 mmHg
Fundus: OD – C:D::0.3:1, foveal reflex is normal; OS – OD – C:D::0.3:1, foveal reflex is dull

1. What is the most probable diagnosis of this condition? 1.______
   A. Macular hole
   B. Central serous retinopathy
   C. Cystoid macular edema
   D. Myopic maculopathy

2. What can be the cause of this condition in the patient? 2.______
   A. Vitreous pulling at the macula
   B. Pulled up pupil
   C. Age of the patient
   D. All of the above

3. Which of the following can be associated with this ocular condition? 3.______
   A. Background diabetic retinopathy
   B. Retinal vein occlusion
   C. Retinitis pigmentosa
   D. All of the above

4. What should we keep looking for in a follow-up of a patient with this disease? 4.______
   - A. Formation of full thickness macular hole
   - B. Formation of lamellar macular hole
   - C. Retinal detachment
   - D. Retinoschisis

5. What are the ophthalmoscopic findings in this condition? 5.______
   - A. Loss of foveal depression
   - B. Thickening of retina
   - C. Multiple cystoid areas
   - D. All of the above

6. What is the level of accumulation of dye in FA in this condition? 6.______
   - A. Outer plexiform layer
   - B. Inner plexiform layer
   - C. Inner nuclear layer
   - D. Outer nuclear layer

7. Where should we look for inflammation in eyes with very little vitreous reaction but significant diminution of vision in patients of this disease? 7.______
   - A. Pars plana
   - B. Optic nerve
   - C. Anterior segment
   - D. Cornea

8. The edema in this condition is restricted to 8.______
   - A. intraretinal
   - B. extraretinal
   - C. intravitreal
   - D. chorioretinal

9. The occurrence of this condition after cataract surgery is known as 9.______
   - A. pars planitis
   - B. Irvine-Gass syndrome
   - C. retinitis
   - D. none of the above

10. The surgical procedure most often associated with this condition is 10.______
    - A. cataract extraction
    - B. filtering procedures for glaucoma
    - C. pars plana vitrectomy
    - D. retinal detachment procedures

Demographics: 40-year-old male
Chief complaint: Diminution of vision in dark and constriction of visual fields
Secondary complaints/symptoms: nil
Patient's ocular history: nil
Patient's medical history: nil
Medications taken by patient: Capsule of Vitamin A for one month last year
Patient's allergy history: Nil
Family ocular history: Father had similar complaints
Family medical history: Nil
Clinical findings: BCVA – OD 6/24; OS – 6/18
Pupils: NSNR in both eyes
Confrontation fields: Constricted in both eyes
Slit lamp: Anterior segment is normal
IOP: 18 mmHg in both eyes
Fundus: Waxy pallor of optic disc in both eyes, bone spicule pigmentation in periphery in fundus, arteriolar attenuation

11. What is the most likely diagnosis of this condition? 11.______

A. Typical retinitis pigmentosa
B. Atypical retinitis pigmentosa
C. Retinitis pigmentosa sine pigmento
D. Retinitis punctata albescens

12. What is the most common mode of inheritance of retinitis pigmentosa? 12.______

A. Autosomal dominant
B. Autosomal recessive
C. X-linked recessive
D. All are equal

13. In typical retinitis pigmentosa, the pigmentary changes are 13.______

A. typically perivascular
B. near optic disc
C. near macula
D. near pars plana

14. The characteristic field defect in typical retinitis pigmentosa is 14.______

A. only peripheral tubular field of vision is left
B. only central field of vision is left
C. arcuate scotoma
D. paracentral scotoma

15. In AD mode of inheritance of RP, clinical manifestations of night blindness and visual field loss develop at 15.______

A. adult life
B. childhood
C. 10 years of age
D. 20 years of age

16. The type of macular lesion described in RP does NOT include 16.______

A. cystoid macular edema
B. atrophic maculopathy
C. cellophane maculopathy
D. central serous retinopathy

17. The associated ocular disease in RP includes 17.______
    A. hypermetropia
    B. retinal detachment
    C. open angle glaucoma
    D. anterior cortical cataract

18. The part of the retina affected in retinitis pigmentosa is 18.______
    A. rods and cones
    B. outer plexiform layer
    C. inner plexiform layer
    D. ganglion cells

19. The differential diagnosis of RP includes 19.______
    A. syphilis
    B. open angle glaucoma
    C. trauma
    D. both A and C

20. Inverse retinitis pigmentosa has pigment distribution 20.______
    A. in the central fundus
    B. at equator
    C. near pars plana
    D. none of the above

21. The electrophysical changes in RP include 21.______
    A. the ERG amplitudes are markedly subnormal
    B. the EOG ratios are substantially abnormal
    C. the ERG latency is increased
    D. all of the above

22. Which of the following is NOT true about retinitis pigmentosa sine pigmento? 22.______
    A. Pigment clumping may ophthalmoscopically absent
    B. Disc atrophy is present
    C. Constricted vessels are present
    D. ERG is normal

23. Which of the following is NOT true about sector retinitis pigmentosa? 23.______
    A. Cases are seen infrequently
    B. Patients may remain asymptomatic for many years
    C. The sector most frequently involved in retina is superior
    D. Typical patients show local fundus changes with constricted retinal vessels

24. The syndrome not associated with RP is 24.______
    A. Marfan's
    B. Bardet-Biedl
    C. Refsum's
    D. Usher's

25. The disease which can produce periphlebitis is 25.______
    A. sarcoidosis
    B. uveitis
    C. syphilis
    D. all of the above

KEY (CORRECT ANSWERS)

1. C
2. A
3. D
4. B
5. D

6. A
7. A
8. A
9. B
10. A

11. A
12. B
13. A
14. B
15. A

16. D
17. C
18. A
19. D
20. A

21. D
22. D
23. C
24. A
25. D

EXAMINATION SECTION

TEST 1

DIRECTIONS: Use the patient information provided to answer the questions that follow. Each question or incomplete statement is followed by several suggested answers or completions. Select the one that BEST answers the question or completes the statement. *PRINT THE LETTER OF THE CORRECT ANSWER IN THE SPACE AT THE RIGHT.*

Demographics: 60-year-old female
Chief complaint: Failure to gain useful vision following cataract surgery in right eye
Secondary complaints/symptoms: Redness, pain, photophobia, diminution of vision and headache
Patient's ocular history: Underwent cataract surgery six weeks ago
Patient's medical history: Patient is diabetic
Medications taken by patient: Systemic antibiotic and analgesic, topical steroids and antibiotics
Patient's allergy history: nil
Family ocular history: nil
Family medical history: nil
Clinical findings: BCVA – OD-6/60; OS-6/9
Pupils: OD – sluggish reaction of pupil to light; OS – pupil NSNR
Confrontation fields: Constricted in right eye, normal in left eye
Slit lamp: OD – Conjunctival congestion, cornea is edematous, mobile hypopyon in anterior chamber, white reflex in pupil; OS – anterior segment is normal
IOP: OD – 16 mmHg; OS – 18 mmHg
Fundus: OD – no glow; OS – within normal limits

1. What is the most probable diagnosis of this condition? 1.______
   A. Bacterial endophthalmitis
   B. Fungal endophthalmitis
   C. Propionobacterium acne endophthalmitis
   D. None of the above

2. What is the most probable causative organism if the onset is delayed? 2.______
   A. Fungal
   B. Staphylococcal epidermidis
   C. Propinobacterium acne
   D. All of the above

3. What is the diagnosis if this case presents additionally with mild restriction of ocular movements? 3.______
   A. Endogenous endophthalmitis
   B. Exogenous endophthalmitis
   C. Panophthalmitis
   D. Extraocular muscle palsy

4. What provides the best specimen for organism identification of this disease? 4.______
   A. Aqueous
   B. Wound margin
   C. Vitreous
   D. Retinal biopsy

5. Which of the following statements is true? 5.______
   A. Aqueous has more ability to resist the infectious agents than vitreous
   B. Vitreous has more ability to resist the infectious agents than aqueous
   C. Both aqueous and vitreous have equal ability to resist infection
   D. None of the above statements are true

6. Which route is preferable to take a vitreous tap? 6.______
   A. Pars plicata route
   B. Pars plana route
   C. Limbal approach
   D. All are equally good

7. The most important treatment step of endophthalmitis is use of __________ antibiotics. 7.______
   A. systemic
   B. subconjunctival
   C. intravitreal
   D. topical

8. What are the indications of vitrectomy in patients with endophthalmitis? 8.______
   A. No improvement of visual acuity or rapid worsening of condition
   B. Suspected fungal endophthalmitis
   C. Retained intraocular foreign body
   D. All of the above

9. Vitrectomy which can be done in patients with endophthalmitis is __________ vitrectomy. 9.______
   A. core
   B. anterior
   C. posterior
   D. total

10. The advantages of vitrectomy include all of the following EXCEPT 10.______
    A. rapid clearance of infection
    B. getting specimen for culture
    C. making better availability of antibiotics
    D. only good for bacterial cases

11. Complications of vitrectomy include all of the following EXCEPT 11.______
    A. cataract formation
    B. rhegmatogenous retinal detachment
    C. tractional retinal detachment
    D. optic neuritis

12. The causative factor for sterile endophthalmitis include all of the following EXCEPT 12.______
    A. undue surgical trauma
    B. incarceration of intraocular contents
    C. fungal infection
    D. use of air and intraocular solution

13. Which antibiotic even by intravenous route reaches the vitreous cavity in sufficient concentrations? 13.______
    A. Ciprofloxacin
    B. Gentamycin
    C. Amikacin
    D. All of the above

14. The precautions needed for giving an intravitreal injection include all of the following EXCEPT: 14.______
    A. Prior to intravitreal injection, do ultrasound to rule out retinal detachment
    B. Bevel of the needle should be anterior
    C. Check IOP of eye before intravitreal injection
    D. Give intravitreal injection in pars plicata region

15. Which of the grading of clarity of ocular media with indirect ophtalmoscopy in patients with endophthalmitis is not correct? 15.______
    A. Grade I – media clarity 6/12, view of retina
    B. Grade II – media clarity < 6/12, can visualize second order retinal vessels
    C. Grade III – vessels not seen, red reflex present
    D. Grade IV – red reflex absent

16. What is the most common presenting symptom of endophthalmitis? 16.______
    A. Blurring of vision
    B. Pain
    C. Photophobia
    D. Any of the above

17. What is the most probable diagnosis if both eyes are affected by this disease? 17.______
    A. Endogenous endophthalmitis
    B. Exogenous endophthalmitis
    C. Endophthalmitis going into panophthalmitis
    D. Orbital cellulites

18. The type of patients included in endophthalmitis vitrectomy study were 18.______
    A. those who had endophthalmitis following trauma
    B. those who had endophthalmitis following cataract surgery
    C. those who had endophthalmitis following fungal infection
    D. all of the above types

19. The intravitreal antibiotics used in intravitreal injection for suspected bacterial endophthalmitis are 19.______
    A. vancomycin and ceftazidime
    B. vancomycin and ciprofloxacin
    C. ciprofloxacin and ceftazidime
    D. ofloxacin and ciprofloxacin

20. The intravitreal antibiotic used in intravitreal injection for suspected fungal endophthalmitis is 20.______
    A. gentamycin
    B. amphotericin B
    C. fluconazole
    D. ketaconazole

Demographics: 55-year-old female
Chief complaint: Painless sudden diminution of vision in right eye – 6 months
Secondary complaints/symptoms: Difficulty seeing central part of field
Patient's ocular history: Nil
Patient's medical history: Nil
Medications taken by patient: Nil
Patient's allergy history: Nil
Family ocular history: Nil
Family medical history: Nil
Clinical findings: BCVA – OD-6/36; OS-6/9
Pupils: OD and OS – NSNR
Confrontation fields: OD and OS normal
Slit lamp: Anterior segment normal in both eyes
IOP: OD – 18 mmHg; OS – 18 mmHg
Fundus: OD – punched out appearance at central fundus, FA – area of hyperfluorescence; OS – within normal limits

21. What is the most probable diagnosis of this condition? 21.______
    A. Senile macular hole
    B. Retinal detachment
    C. Vitreous hemorrhage
    D. Diabetic retinopathy

22. What type of visual loss is present in this condition? 22.______
    A. Full field defect
    B. Central vision loss
    C. Peripheral visual loss
    D. Any of the above

23. What is Watzke-Allen sign in patients with macular hole? 23.______
    A. Break or thinning of the slit lamp beam in macular region
    B. Elevation of retina at macula
    C. Oedema of retina at macula
    D. Foreign body at macula

24. How does a macular hole enlarge? 24.______
    A. Persistent tangential traction from the vitreous
    B. Tangential traction from the epiretinal membrane
    C. Development of large cystic spaces within the surrounding cuff
    D. All of the above

25. What are the lesions that can mimic a macular hole? 25.______
    A. An epiretinal membrane with a pseudohole
    B. A foveal detachment due to central serous retinopathy
    C. Cystoid macular edema
    D. Any of the above

26. How is the full thickness hole most accurately diagnosed clinically? 26.______
    A. With a fundus contact lens and slit lamp biomicroscopy
    B. Direct ophthalmoscopy
    C. Indirect ophthalmoscopy
    D. Hruby lens

27. How can cystoid macular edema be differentiated from a macula hole? 27.______
    A. Fluorescein angiography
    B. History of cataract extraction
    C. Examination with fundus contact lens and slit lamp biomicroscopy
    D. All of the above

28. How can the absolute and relative scotomas associated with macular hole be analyzed? 28.______
    A. Microperimetry with scanning laser ophthalmoscope
    B. Humphrey field analyzer
    C. Goldman perimetry
    D. Confrontation perimetry

29. The disease entities which optical coherence tomography can diagnose in the macular region are 29.______
    A. full thickness holes
    B. partial thickness holes
    C. macular cyst
    D. all of the above

30. Which of the following statements is incorrect? 30.______
    A. Gradual sloping margins with irregular edges characterize degenerative hole of recent origin
    B. The sloping borders of hole become well defined usually over a period of four months
    C. Undermining of retinal edges is the first phenomenon in formation of macular hole
    D. The classic macular hole is a round excavation with sharply punched out margins

KEY (CORRECT ANSWERS)

1. A	11. D	21. A
2. D	12. C	22. B
3. C	13. A	23. A
4. C	14. D	24. D
5. A	15. C	25. D
6. B	16. A	26. A
7. C	17. A	27. D
8. D	18. B	28. A
9. A	19. A	29. D
10. D	20. B	30. C

TEST 2

DIRECTIONS: Use the patient information provided to answer the questions that follow. Each question or incomplete statement is followed by several suggested answers or completions. Select the one that BEST answers the question or completes the statement. *PRINT THE LETTER OF THE CORRECT ANSWER IN THE SPACE AT THE RIGHT.*

1. The most common form of macular hole is 1.______
   A. traumatic
   B. senile macular hole in elderly women
   C. myopia
   D. solar retinopathy

2. A pseudohole is different from macular hole in all of these ways EXCEPT: 2.______
   A. Has worse vision than does a macular hole
   B. Does not have halo of fluid
   C. Does not have operculum
   D. Does not have yellow deposits at level of RPE

3. Which of the following statements is false? 3.______
   A. Occurrence of retinal detachment in patient with macular hole is quite common
   B. Retinal detachment occurs in patients with macular hole if the patient is high myope
   C. Retinal detachment occurs in patients with macular hole if the patient experiences ocular trauma
   D. None of the above

Demographics: 25-year-old female
Chief complaint: Diminution of vision in both eyes, appearance of multiple images monocularly for five years
Secondary complaints/symptoms: A cone-like projection in central cornea in both eyes
Patient's ocular history: Diminution of vision since childhood
Patient's medical history: Nil
Medications taken by patient: Nil
Patient's allergy history: nil
Family ocular history: A brother had similar complaint
Family medical history: nil
Clinical findings: BCVA – OD-6/12; OS-6/18
Pupils: OD and OS NSNR
Confrontation fields: OD and OS normal
Slit lamp: A cone-like projection in both eyes in central cornea, a brown line is observed at the base of cone when examined in slit lamp red free light
IOP: OD – 16 mmHg; OS – 16 mmHg
Fundus: OD – within normal limits

4. What is the most likely diagnosis of this condition? 4.______
   A. Anterior staphyloma
   B. Phthisis bulbi
   C. Keratoconus
   D. Mooren's ulcer

5. What is the most probable cause of this disease? 5.______
   A. Inflammation
   B. Trauma
   C. Surgery
   D. None of the above

6. Which other ocular abnormality would you expect in this patient? 6.______
   A. Retinitis pigmentosa
   B. Down's syndrome
   C. Vernal keratoconjunctivitis
   D. All of the above

7. Which systemic diseases can be found in this patient? 7.______
   I. Marfan's syndrome
   II. Ehler's Danlos syndrome
   III. Thyroid disease
   IV. Addison's disease

   A. I only B. I and II C. I, II and III D. I, II, III, IV

8. Which enzyme abnormality is found in epithelium of keratoconus patient? 8.______
   A. Glucose 6 phosphate dehydrogenase
   B. Lactate dehydrogenase
   C. Fructokinase
   D. Galactokinase

9. What is the name given to the brown line around the base of the cone? 9.______
   A. Fleischer's ring
   B. Kayser-Fleischer's ring
   C. Stoker's line
   D. Fleiringa's ring

10. The angular appearance of lower eyelid margin conforming to curvature of cone in such patient is 10.______
    A. Munson's sign
    B. acute hydrops
    C. distichiasis
    D. mechanical ectropion

11. What is the expected refractive error in this patient? 11.______
    A. Regular myopic astigmatism
    B. Regular hypermetropic astigmatism
    C. Irregular myopic astigmatism
    D. Any of the above

12. What cannot be the keratometric finding in this patient? 12.______
    A. High cylinders at oblique axis
    B. Mires will be grossly irregular
    C. K reading may become so high to be measured on the usual scale
    D. Viewing the cornea through photoelectric keratometer will not exhibit gross distortion of rings

13. The diagnostic sign for this condition does NOT include 13.______
    A. increased corneal sensation at apex of cone
    B. vertical stress lines or Vogt's bands seen in the deep stroma and Descemet's membrane at the apex of cone
    C. prominent corneal nerves
    D. brown ring consisting of iron pigment in the deep epithelium around the base of cone

14. The clinical features of acute hydrops in this patient does NOT include 14.______
    A. sudden onset of blurred vision
    B. grossly clouded cornea
    C. more frequent occurrence in patients with Down's syndrome
    D. the hydropic cornea finally perforates in all patients

15. What is the dystrophy in which non-inflammatory thinning of cornea occurs in periphery of cornea which gradually progresses toward center? 15.______
    A. Keratoglobus
    B. Terrien's marginal degeneration
    C. Mooren's ulcer
    D. Dellen

16. Which feature differentiates the hydrops which occurs in keratoglobus from that which occurs in keratoconus? 16.______
    A. It is much more likely to become vascularised as it heals
    B. The hydrops of keratoglobus leads to perforation more frequently
    C. In keratoglobus, hydrops starts in center and proceeds toward periphery
    D. None of the above

17. The differences between keratoglobus and keratoconus do NOT include 17.______
    A. keratoglobus is more rare
    B. there is irregular myopic astigmatism in keratoconus but not in keratoglobus
    C. keratoglobus begins in periphery while keratoconus begins in center
    D. it is extremely difficult to fit a patient of keratoglobus with contact lens while it is not so in patient with keratoconus

Demographics: 55-year-old male
Chief complaint: Sudden profound painful diminution of vision in right eye – 1 week
Secondary complaints/symptoms: Nil
Patient's ocular history: Nil
Patient's medical history: Nil
Medications taken by patient: Nil
Patient's allergy history: nil
Family ocular history: Nil
Family medical history: nil
Clinical findings: BCVA – OD-6/60; OS-6/6
Pupils: OD – dilated pupil with sluggish reaction to light; OS – NSNR
Confrontation fields: OD – central scotoma; OS – normal
Slit lamp: Anterior segment in both eyes – normal
IOP: OD – 18 mmHg; OS – 18 mmHg
Fundus: OD – Hyperemic optic disc with blurring of margins, oedema of optic disc with obliteration of optic cup, foveal reflex normal; OS within normal limits

18. What is the most likely diagnosis of this condition? 18.______
    A. Optic neuritis
    B. Central retinal vein occlusion
    C. Central retinal artery occlusion
    D. Papilledema

19. What is the most likely site of affection if the fundus findings are normal while the rest of the clinical presentation remains the same? 19.______
    A. Optic nerve head
    B. Retrobulbar region
    C. Anterior segment
    D. Corneal

20. The sign which indicates worsening of impairment of vision with rise of body temperature is __________ sign. 20.______
    A. Uthoff's
    B. Munson's
    C. Hutchison's
    D. Kocher's

21. Which is the most likely cause of pain associated with movement of the eyeball in this patient? 21.______
    A. Spread of infection to eyelids
    B. Associated orbital cellulites
    C. Spread of inflammation to superior rectus
    D. Associated cavernous sinus thrombosis

22. The other clinical signs which can be found in this condition include all of the following EXCEPT 22.______
    A. severe impairment of color vision in affected eye
    B. lowered dark adaptation in affected eye
    C. afferent pupillary defect in affected eye
    D. tenderness on palpation of the globe is always present

23. What is the name of the condition in which the appearance of the optic disc is the same as it is found in this patient? 23.______
    A. Papilledema
    B. Pseudopapillitis
    C. Chorioretinitis
    D. None of the above

24. Which aetiological factor can possibly cause this ocular disease? 24.______
    A. Idiopathic
    B. Demyelinating disease
    C. Viral infection
    D. All of the above

25. Which of the following is false regarding idiopathic stellate maculopathy? 25.______
    A. It has all the features of optic neuritis
    B. There is a macular star
    C. It is associated with multiple sclerosis
    D. It is an uncommon manifestation (in patients of optic neuritis) as compared to papillitis

26. The toxic degenerative optic neuritis can be caused by 26.______
    A. tobacco
    B. methyl alcohol
    C. lead
    D. all of the above

27. The clinical feature which is not true for temporal arteritis is 27.______
    A. it is one of the significant causes of ischemic optic neuritis
    B. the ESR is not raised
    C. there is polymyalgia rheumatica
    D. there are tender beaded and tortuous temporal arteries

28. Which is true of Pulfrich's phenomenon? 28.______
    A. It is due to difference in conduction of impulses from two eyes
    B. In normal eye, a pendulum swinging in a frontal plane is seen as though it were moving along an elliptical if a neutral density filter is placed in front of one eye
    C. This phenomenon will not occur in patients with severe degree of visual impairment
    D. All of the above

29. Uhthoff's symptoms can occur 29.______
    A. in isolated optic neuritis
    B. in multiple sclerosis
    C. due to exposure to hot baths or showers in patient of optic neuritis
    D. all of the above

30. Uhthoff's symptom in multiple sclerosis cannot be detected by 30.______
    A. changes in contrast sensitivity
    B. slit lamp examination on anterior segment
    C. fluctuation in VEP amplitude
    D. Farnsworth Munsell 100 hue testing

KEY (CORRECT ANSWERS)

1. B	11. C	21. C
2. A	12. D	22. D
3. A	13. A	23. B
4. C	14. D	24. D
5. D	15. A	25. C
6. D	16. A	26. D
7. D	17. B	27. B
8. A	18. A	28. D
9. A	19. B	29. D
10. A	20. A	30. B

TEST 3

DIRECTIONS: Use the patient information provided to answer the questions that follow. Each question or incomplete statement is followed by several suggested answers or completions. Select the one that BEST answers the question or completes the statement. *PRINT THE LETTER OF THE CORRECT ANSWER IN THE SPACE AT THE RIGHT.*

1. What is not the usual cause for simultaneous or sequential bilateral optic neuritis? 1.______
   A. Devic's disease
   B. Immune mediated optic neuropathy
   C. Idiopathic optic neuritis
   D. Nutritional amblyopia

2. The Leber's hereditary optic neuritis is characterized by all of the following features EXCEPT 2.______
   A. it is maternally inherited
   B. primarily affects females
   C. there are central or cecocentral scotoma
   D. fluorescein fundus angiography does not show any evidence of abnormal vascular permeability

3. The inheritance pattern for Leber's hereditary optic neuropathy is 3.______
   A. autosomal recessive
   B. autosomal dominant
   C. inherited mutations in mitochondrial DNA
   D. sporadic

4. Which of the following is true of pattern VEP? 4.______
   A. Tests central and perifoveal visual field
   B. It is generated in cortical area 17, 18, 19
   C. The only positive component of waveform is P 100
   D. All of the above

5. Which of the following is NOT true of Behr's hereditary optic atrophy? 5.______
   A. Begins in young age
   B. The visual loss stabilizes by 2nd or 3rd decade
   C. It is transmitted as an AR trait
   D. It may be associated with neurological abnormality like cerebellar ataxia

6. The antitubercular drugs which can cause optic neuritis are 6.______
   A. ethambutol and isoniazide
   B. isoniazide and rifampicin
   C. ethambutol and rifampicin
   D. all of the above

Demographics: 50-year-old male
Chief complaint: Small ulcer on left lower lid near medial canthus – one year; it is very slowly growing in size
Secondary complaints/symptoms: Occasional watery discharge from lesion
Patient's ocular history: Patient was operated for cataract in right eye; has cataract in left eye
Patient's medical history: Nil
Medications taken by patient: Nil
Patient's allergy history: nil
Family ocular history: Nil
Family medical history: nil
Clinical findings: BCVA – OD-6/9; OS-6/36
Pupils: OD and OS – NSNR
Confrontation fields: OD and OS – normal
Slit lamp: Anterior segment in both eyes – normal
IOP: OD – 16 mmHg; OS – 16 mmHg
Fundus: OD and OS – C:D::0.3:1, foveal reflex normal
Local study: Solid type of lesion with central ulceration and indurated base, some telangectasia are present

7. What is the most likely diagnosis of this condition? 7.______
   A. Basal cell carcinoma
   B. Squamous cell carcinoma
   C. Chalazion
   D. Hordeolum internum

8. Which is the most common malignant tumor of eyelids? 8.______
   A. Basal cell carcinoma
   B. Squamous cell carcinoma
   C. Lacrimal sac tumor
   D. Adenocarcinoma

9. Which lid carcinoma has metastasis through lymphatics? 9.______
   I. Basal cell carcinoma
   II. Squamous cell carcinoma
   III. Adenocarcinoma
   IV. Keratoacanthoma

   A. Only I
   B. Only II
   C. II and III
   D. Only IV

10. In which lid is a chalazion more common? 10.______
    A. Equal in both lids
    B. More in upper lid
    C. More in lower lid
    D. No such predilection noted

11. Multiple chalazions are found in association with 11.______
    A. seborrhea
    B. chronic blepharitis
    C. acne rosacea
    D. all of the above

12. Which is not considered the modality of treatment for chalazion? 12.______
    A. Hot fomentation
    B. Incision and curettage
    C. Intralesional therapy of triamcinolone
    D. Radiation therapy

13. Which statement is NOT correct? 13.______
    A. Hordeolum internum is inflammation of mebomian glands and hordeolum externum is inflammation of the Ziess gland
    B. Hordeolum internum is more painful than hordeolum externum
    C. An abscess in hordeolum externum points near the base of one of the cilia while in hordeolum internum, it appears as a yellow spot shining through conjunctiva
    D. Both hordeolum internum and hordeolum externum may be due to secondary infection of chalazion

14. Which of the following statements is false? 14.______
    A. Basal cell carcinoma is locally invasive
    B. Squamous cell carcinoma is painful if there is involvement of nerves
    C. Surgery is recommended for extensive carcinoma
    D. Keratin pearls are found in squamous cell carcinoma

15. The carcinoma which involves mebomian gland is called 15.______
    A. Basal cell carcinoma
    B. Squamous cell carcinoma
    C. Adenocarcinoma
    D. Keratoacanthoma

16. Which is not true of an adenocarcinoma? 16.______
    A. Appears like hard chalazion
    B. Has several inflammatory signs in elderly persons
    C. May have presentation like tarsitis, ulceration of lid margin, atrophy of skin of lid margin
    D. If suspicion is there, chalazion should be totally excised and subjected to histopathology

17. The prognosis for which site of basal cell carcinoma is worst? 17.______
    A. On lower lid
    B. On upper lid
    C. AT inner canthus
    D. All have same prognosis

18. What histopathology does not characterize basal cell carcinoma? 18.______
    A. The cells resemble basal cells
    B. The nuclei of these cells stain deeply basophilic giving tumor a discretely dark blue appearance on staining with hematoxylin and eosin
    C. Peripheral palisading of basal cells is characteristic
    D. Keratin pearls are visible on section

Demographics: 40-year-old male
Chief complaint: Bilateral herpes zoster ophthalmicus with severe involvement of skin and ectropion of eyelids with it
Secondary complaints/symptoms: Foreign body sensation, pain, redness, watering and diminution of vision in both eyes
Patient's ocular history: Not significant
Patient's medical history: Patient is homosexual – he has been having fever, weight loss, generalized lymphadenopathy for three months
Medications taken by patient: Zidovudine
Patient's allergy history: nil
Family ocular history: Nil
Family medical history: nil
Clinical findings: BCVA – OD-6/24; OS-6/18
Pupils: OD and OS – NSNR
Confrontation fields: OD and OS – appear normal
Slit lamp: Amoeboid corneal ulcer in both eyes involving stromal region and a few keratic precipitates are present
IOP: Not possible to take in present setting
Fundus: Not possible to examine due to media opacity

19. What is the most likely disease the patient is suffering from? 19.______
    A. AIDS
    B. Severe herpes zoster ophthalmicus
    C. Bilateral herpes zoster ophthalmicus
    D. None of the above

20. The principle modes of transmission of this virus include all EXCEPT 20.______
    A. vaginal and anal intercourse between male and female
    B. transfusion of infected blood
    C. injection with non-sterile needle
    D. hugging an infected patient

21. Maternal-infant transmission of this virus can take place 21.______
    A. perinatally in utero
    B. perinatally during delivery
    C. during breast feeding
    D. all of the above

22. The vaccines which can be given to all asymptomatic infected children (with virus) are 22.______
    A. all standard vaccines – both live and attenuated
    B. live vaccines only
    C. attenuated vaccines only
    D. no vaccine should be given

23. What cannot be found in the retina of this patient? 23._______
    A. Cotton wool spots
    B. Drusens
    C. CMV retinitis
    D. Retinal perivasculutis

24. Which of the following tests is not useful for detecting HIV infection in children less than seven months of age? 24._______
    A. ELISA
    B. Viral culture
    C. Polymerase chain reaction
    D. Detection of p 24 antigen in serum

25. In which group of people is AIDS testing not mandatory? 25._______
    A. Blood donors
    B. Organ donors
    C. All hospital personnel
    D. Overseas student

26. HIV can be isolated from which ocular structure? 26._______
    A. Tears
    B. Cornea
    C. Aqueous humor
    D. All of the above

27. CMV retinitis is the most common AIDS related infection at CD4 counts 27._______
    A. < 200/mm3
    B. < 100/mm3
    C. < 50/mm3
    D. All of these

28. What picture would a patient with AIDS be advised to check for the appearance of CMV retinitis? 28._______
    A. Development of peripheral or central scotoma
    B. Appearance of extraocular muscle palsy
    C. Appearance of color blindness
    D. All of the above

29. What drug is not advocated for management of patient with AIDS? 29._______
    A. Gancyclovir
    B. Foscarnet
    C. Rifampicin
    D. Zidovudine

30. The neoplasm which is common in patients with AIDS is 30._______
    A. Kaposi sarcoma
    B. squamous cell carcinoma
    C. basal cell carcinoma
    D. all of the above

31. How will you take IOP in this patient? 31._______
    A. Mackay-Marg tonometer
    B. Maklakov tonometer
    C. Canon TX-10 non-contact tonometer
    D. Perkin's handheld tonometer

32. What are the serious complications which should be looked out for in this patient? 32.______
    A. CMV retinitis
    B. Progressive outer retinal necrosis
    C. Bilateral corneal opacities and ulcers
    D. All of the above

33. What precautions would you not observe while doing lid surgery for correction in this patient? 33.______
    A. Use double gloving
    B. Avoid needle pricks
    C. Use zidovudine/lamivudine in case of needle pricks
    D. Avoid oozing of blood from wound

34. Which of the following is NOT associated with subretinal neovascular membrane? 34.______
    A. Choroidal rupture
    B. Best's disease
    C. Rubella retinopathy
    D. Severe hypermetropia

35. Hyperfluorescence in fluoroscein angiography cannot be due to 35.______
    A. increased quantity of extravascular fluoroscein leakage into serous or hemorrhagic areas
    B. drusens
    C. decrease in the filter effect of pigment epithelium
    D. vascular tumors

KEY (CORRECT ANSWERS)

1. C	11. D	21. D	31. C
2. B	12. D	22. A	32. D
3. C	13. D	23. B	33. D
4. D	14. C	24. A	34. D
5. A	15. C	25. D	35. D
6. A	16. B	26. D	
7. A	17. C	27. C	
8. A	18. D	28. A	
9. C	19. A	29. C	
10. B	20. D	30. A	

EXAMINATION SECTION

TEST 1

DIRECTIONS: Use the patient information provided to answer the questions that follow. Each question or incomplete statement is followed by several suggested answers or completions. Select the one that BEST answers the question or completes the statement. *PRINT THE LETTER OF THE CORRECT ANSWER IN THE SPACE AT THE RIGHT.*

Demographics: 40-year-old male
Chief complaint: Diminution of vision from corneal opacity in both eyes
Secondary complaints/symptoms: Foreign body sensation in both eyes, mild redness in both eyes, dryness in both eyes
Patient's ocular history: Patient had corneal ulcer in both eyes – two years ago
Patient's medical history: Patient is diabetic
Medications taken by patient: Topical artificial tears
Patient's allergy history: nil
Family ocular history: nil
Family medical history: nil
Clinical findings: BCVA – OD 6/60; OS 6/24
Pupils: OD and OS – NSNR
Confrontation fields: Constricted in both eyes
Slit lamp: OD-OS – corneal opacity extending through all layers of cornea in both eyes, lens clear, no evidence of uveitis
IOP: OD – 16 mmHg; OS – 18 mmHg
Fundus: OD-OS – in dilated pupil – C:D::0.3:1, foveal reflex normal

1. What is the most likely cause of corneal opacity in this patient? 1.______
   A. Diabetes B. Herpes keratitis
   C. Dry eyes D. Nutritional

2. Which tonometer would you prefer to take IOP in his eyes? 2.______
   A. Mackay Marg B. Maklakov
   C. Schiotz D. Perkins

3. What is the most appropriate treatment you would advise this patient based on clinical finding? 3.______
   A. Penetrating keratoplasty B. Lamellar keratoplasty
   C. Contact lenses D. Glasses

4. What investigations would you not order if you take this patient for keratoplasty? 4.______
   A. Tonometry B. USB B scan
   C. Focal VEP D. X-ray orbit AP and lateral view

5. What would you test the blood for before you take the patient for keratoplasty? 5.______
   A. Hepatitis B. HIV C. Rabies D. All of these

6. What cannot be a cause for bilateral corneal opacity in a patient of this age? 6.______
   A. Stevens Johnson syndrome B. Keratoconus
   C. Chemical burns D. Diabetes

7. If the posterior and anterior segments of both eyes are normal, which eye in this patient would you take for keratoplasty first? 7.______
   A. Right eye B. Left eye
   C. Either eye D. No way to determine

8. With which instrument would you see the fundus in this patient? 8.______
   A. Direct ophthalmoscope
   B. Indirect ophthalmoscope
   C. Hruby lens
   D. Fundus contact lens

9. What can be the sequalae of corneal opacity in this patient? 9.______
   A. Amblyopia B. Complicated cataract
   C. Uveitis D. None of the above

10. Which corneal opacity is more deleterious to vision? 10.______
   A. Central nebular opacity
   B. Peripheral macular opacity
   C. Peripheral leucomatous opacity
   D. All are equally deleterious to vision

Demographics: 60-year-old male
Chief complaint: Needs glasses for both eyes, which have been operated for cataract without IOL implantation
Secondary complaints/symptoms: Pain, redness, watering in both eyes; has a lot of visual inconvenience present like difficulty in climbing stairs, pouring water onto table instead if into glass, etc.
Patient's ocular history: As given before
Patient's medical history: nil
Medications taken by patient: nil
Patient's allergy history: nil
Family ocular history: nil
Family medical history: nil
Clinical findings: BCVA – OD 6/24; OS 6/24
Pupils: OD and OS – NSNR
Hirshberg test: Orthophoria
Confrontation fields: Appear normal
Slit lamp: OD-OS – Absence of lens from pupillary area
IOP: OD – 16 mmHg; OS – 18 mmHg
Gonioscopy: Open anterior chamber angle with broad ciliary band
Fundus: OD-OS – small optic disc, C:D::0.3:1, foveal reflex normal

11. What is the probable diagnosis for both eyes? 11.______
    A. Pseudophakia B. Aphakia
    C. Cataract D. None of the above

12. What is the pupillary reflex like in patient who has cataract operated without IOL implantation? 12.______
    A. Grey B. Silver
    C. Jet black D. White

13. What problem can this patient face without the use of appropriate glasses? 13.______
    A. Suppression in operated eye (when only one eye was operated)
    B. Lack of fusion
    C. Poor visual acuity
    D. All of the above

14. What problem can this patient face with the use of appropriate glasses? 14.______
    A. Roving scotoma
    B. Jack-in-box phenomenon
    C. Pin cushion effect
    D. All of the above

15. Which Purkinje-Samson image would be missing in this patient? 15.______
    A. 1 & 2 B. 2 & 3 C. 3 & 4 D. 1 & 4

16. The intraocular pressure in this patient would be __________ the normal control subject of the same age. 16.______
    A. less than
    B. same as
    C. more than
    D. any of the above

17. What would be the apparent size of optic disc when seen with direct ophthalmoscopy in this patient? 17.______
    A. Appears smaller than it actually is
    B. Appears larger than it actually is
    C. Appears of the same size
    D. Any of the above

18. The contact element in Goldman applanation tonometer is 18.______
    A. prism with apex upwards
    B. biprisms
    C. prism with apex downwards
    D. convex lens

19. The mirror in the Goldman gonioscope is inclined at what angle to the flat surface? 19.______
    A. 64° B. 62° C. 54° D. 47°

20. In this patient, with use of direct ophthalmoscopy, the field of vision of the examiner in the patient's eye will be __________ that seen in a normal emmetropic person. 20.______
    A. greater than
    B. same as
    C. smaller than
    D. any of the above

21. In a preliminary examination of the patient's eye at 1m distance from the examiner, with light source and plane mirror of the Priestly-Smith retinoscope, what would be seen in the pupil? 21.______
    A. Uniform red glow
    B. Hazy image of the fundus
    C. Uniform dark glow
    D. None of the above

22. The formula for calculation of refractive power of an eye is: Refractive error equals 22.______
    A. 100/PR + 3, PR is the punctum remotum
    B. 100/PR – 3
    C. PR + 3 / 100
    D. PR – 3 / 100

23. While doing retinoscopy in this patient's eye using the plane mirror, movement of the illuminated spot on fundus will be 23.______
    A. in same direction as the movement of mirror
    B. in opposite direction as the movement of mirror
    C. can be either of the above depending on degree of accommodation
    D. plane mirror is not used in retinoscopy

24. While doing retinoscopy in this patient's eye using concave mirror, the movement of the illuminated spot on fundus will be 24.______
    A. in same direction as that of mirror
    B. in opposite direction as that of mirror
    C. can be in either direction depending on accommodation by patient
    D. none of the above

25. In this patient's eye, the position of the nodal points would shift in which direction? 25.______
    A. Two nodal points shift backward
    B. First nodal point shifts forward
    C. Second nodal point shifts backward
    D. Both nodal points shift forward

KEY (CORRECT ANSWERS)

1. B	11. B	21. B
2. A	12. C	22. A
3. A	13. C	23. A
4. D	14. D	24. B
5. D	15. C	25. D
6. D	16. D	
7. A	17. A	
8. B	18. B	
9. D	19. A	
10. A	20. A	

TEST 2

DIRECTIONS: Use the patient information provided to answer the questions that follow. Each question or incomplete statement is followed by several suggested answers or completions. Select the one that BEST answers the question or completes the statement. *PRINT THE LETTER OF THE CORRECT ANSWER IN THE SPACE AT THE RIGHT.*

Demographics: 60-year-old male
Chief complaint: Needs glasses for both eyes, which have been operated for cataract without IOL implantation
Secondary complaints/symptoms: Pain, redness, watering in both eyes; has a lot of visual inconvenience present like difficulty in climbing stairs, pouring water onto table instead if into glass, etc.
Patient's ocular history: As given before
Patient's medical history: nil
Medications taken by patient: nil
Patient's allergy history: nil
Family ocular history: nil
Family medical history: nil
Clinical findings: BCVA – OD 6/24; OS 6/24
Pupils: OD and OS – NSNR
Hirshberg test: Orthophoria
Confrontation fields: Appear normal
Slit lamp: OD-OS – Absence of lens from pupillary area
IOP: OD – 16 mmHg; OS – 18 mmHg
Gonioscopy: Open anterior chamber angle with broad ciliary band
Fundus: OD-OS – small optic disc, C:D::0.3:1, foveal reflex normal

1. The image in this eye, after refractive correction is worn at anterior focal distance, will be larger than the emmetropic eye by what factor? 1.______
   A. 1/3 B. 1/4 C. 1/2 D. 1/5

2. In this patient, when we record the vision on Snellen's chart, the vision recorded is 2.______
   A. better than the actual visual acuity
   B. worse than the actual visual acuity
   C. same as the actual visual acuity
   D. any of the above depending on the illumination condition of the room

3. The pin cushion distortion in this patient is caused by 3.______
   A. chromatic aberration B. spherical aberration
   C. sine condition D. refraction by eccentric rays

4. The expected useful monocular and binocular of vision in this patient is about ______ all round. 4.______
   A. 180° B. 150° C. 120° D. 50°

5. The characteristics of ring scotoma in front of this patient's eye include all of the following EXCEPT 5.______
   A. the ring scotoma is 15° in size
   B. it is caused by the prismatic effect at the periphery of the correcting lens
   C. the scotoma tends to move with an against motion to the motion of the eye
   D. as the eye moves to the peripheral lens position, the scotoma also moves to the more peripheral position

6. Which is not true about determination of refractive error in this patient? 6.______
   A. Keratometric readings are valuable because astigmatism is entirely corneal
   B. The pupil can be dilated with phenylepherine
   C. Cycloplegia is a must
   D. In retinoscopy, the shadow is faint and it moves with the movement of mirror using plane mirror in retinoscope

7. Which is not true about binocular vision in this patient? 7.______
   A. Even in binocular aphakia, binocularity is not always present
   B. Binocularity in unilateral aphakia is easy to achieve
   C. If binocularity has existed before in life, it can be restored after cataract removal in both eyes
   D. It is unwise to fix the operation of the second eye in bilateral cataracts after a long time, i.e. the inter-operation interval should not be long

8. The major hindrance to binocularity in this patient when he is uniocularly operated is difference in the size of image formed by two eyes, which is about 8.______
   A. 10% B. 20% C. 30% D. 40%

9. Which statement is not true regarding aniseikonia in this patient (when only one eye was operated for cataract extraction)? 9.______
   A. Aniseikonia with spectacle glasses placed 15 mm in front of cornea is about 30%
   B. Aniseikonia with contact lenses used is about 10-13%
   C. Aniseikonia with Strampelli's anterior chamber implant is 5%
   D. Aniseikonia with Ridley type posterior chamber implant is 2%

10. What are the advantages of contact lens use in this patient? 10.______
    A. Less aniseikonia
    B. Elimination of various aberrations and prismatic effect of spectacle glasses
    C. Eyes can move more freely as the relative position of contact lenses remains constant
    D. All of the above

11. Which problem cannot be solved even with the use of IOL in this patient? 11.______
    A. Magnification defects are reduced
    B. Phenomenon like jack-in-box is totally eliminated
    C. Accommodation is restored
    D. Phenomenon of pin cushion distortion is eliminated

12. The causes of astigmatism in this patient following lens extraction can be related to which of the following factors? 12.______
    A. Size and material of sutures used
    B. Tightness of sutures
    C. Size of wound and nearness to the cornea
    D. All of the above

13. The parallel rays of light would come to focus in this patient at ______ mm behind the cornea. 13.______
    A. 5   B. 17   C. 23   D. 31

14. For what reason could this patient experience visual incoordination, like pouring water onto the table instead of into a glass? 14.______
    A. Relative magnification due to removal of lens introduces a false spatial orientation of objects
    B. Due to prismatic effect caused by absence of lens
    C. Due to spherical aberration caused by absence of lens
    D. Due to chromatic aberration caused by absence of lens

15. What can be the cause of visual problems that a secondary IOL implantation can lead to in this patient? 15.______
    A. Eccentration of IOL
    B. Tilt of IOL
    C. Lens edge or dialing hole opposite to the pupil
    D. All of the above

16. Which of the following is an ocular complication that this patient is likely to face due to absence of lens? 16.______
    A. Endodonesis   B. Retinal detachment
    C. Cystoid macular edema   D. All of the above

4 (#2)

Demographics: 10-year-old female
Chief complaint: Difficulty in seeing near objects
Secondary complaints/symptoms: Strain, headache on doing prolonged near work
Patient's ocular history: nil
Patient's medical history: nil
Medications taken by patient: After doing cycloplegic refraction it was found that she was corrected with +3.0 Dsph in both eyes to 6/5
Patient's allergy history: nil
Family ocular history: Elder sister had similar complaints and was corrected by using glasses
Family medical history: nil
Clinical findings: BCVA – OD 6/5 with pin hole; OS – 6/5 with pin hole
Pupils: OD and OS – NSNR
Hirshberg test: Orthophoria
Confrontation fields: Appear normal in both eyes
Slit lamp: OD-OS – Anterior segment is normal
IOP: OD – 18 mmHg; OS – 18 mmHg
Fundus: OD-OS – small optic disc, C:D::0.3:1, foveal reflex normal

17. What is the most likely diagnosis of this condition? 17.______
    A. Myopia
    B. Hypermetropia
    C. Presbyopia
    D. Astigmatism

18. Where is the posterior principal focus of the eye situated in this patient? 18.______
    A. Posterior to retinal plane
    B. On retinal plane
    C. Anterior to retinal plane
    D. In mid-vitreous

19. When dry refraction (without cycloplegia) was done, the error of hypermetropia was found only +2.0 Dsph in both eyes while with cycloplegia, total error was found +3.0 Dsph. Hence, in this patient, +1.0 Dsph is __________ hypermetropia. 19.______
    A. facultative
    B. latent
    C. absolute
    D. manifest

20. Which investigation is not indicated to rule out pathological hypermetropia? 20.______
    A. Axial length
    B. Keratometry
    C. Indirect ophthalmoscopy
    D. Fluorescein angiography

21. Which method would you use to find the facultative hypermetropia in this patient? 21.______
    A. Complete cycloplegia
    B. Ask the patient to look at distance
    C. Fogging method
    D. Use of phenylepherine

22. A change in refractive error that would take place once this patient reaches about 50 years of age is 22.______
    A. the refractive error will become of index type
    B. the refractive error will become increasingly absolute
    C. facultative and latent part will become less
    D. all of the above

23. Which of the following is a disease this patient can have in association with this refractive error? 23.______
    A. Convergent strabismus
    B. Angle closure glaucoma
    C. Amblyopia
    D. All of the above

24. What would be the change in degree of refractive error if the eyeball is 2 mm shorter than normal? 24.______
    A. 6 D
    B. 3 D
    C. 4 D
    D. 5 D

25. Which fundus finding is not expected in this patient? 25.______
    A. Shot silk retina
    B. Papilledema like optic disc
    C. Macula is situated further from the disc than is usual in emmetropic eye
    D. Pseudopapillitis

KEY (CORRECT ANSWERS)

1. A	11. C	21. C
2. A	12. D	22. D
3. B	13. D	23. D
4. D	14. A	24. A
5. D	15. D	25. B
6. C	16. D	
7. B	17. B	
8. C	18. A	
9. D	19. B	
10. D	20. D	

TEST 3

DIRECTIONS: Use the patient information provided to answer the questions that follow. Each question or incomplete statement is followed by several suggested answers or completions. Select the one that BEST answers the question or completes the statement. *PRINT THE LETTER OF THE CORRECT ANSWER IN THE SPACE AT THE RIGHT.*

Demographics: 9-year-old male
Chief complaint: Difficulty seeing distant objects – he has to half close his lids when looking at blackboard to read; does not prefer outdoor sports
Secondary complaints/symptoms: Redness and watering in both eyes very frequently
Patient's ocular history: Never used any spectacles before
Patient's medical history: nil
Medications taken by patient: nil
Patient's allergy history: nil
Family ocular history: nil
Family medical history: nil
Clinical findings: BCVA – OD 6/5; OS 6/5 with – 6.0 D lens in both eyes
Pupils: OD and OS – NSNR
Hirshberg test: Orthophoria
Confrontation fields: Appear normal
Slit lamp: OD-OS – Anterior segment is normal
IOP: OD – 16 mmHg; OS – 16 mmHg
Fundus: OD-OS – large optic disc, C:D::0.3:1, foveal reflex normal

1. What is the most likely diagnosis of this condition? 1.______
   A. Myopia
   B. Hypermetropia
   C. Presbyopia
   D. Astigmatism

2. The punctum remotum (in meters) of this eye is given as 2.______
   A. reciprocal of the diopteric value of its refractive error
   B. diopteric value of its refractive error
   C. range of accommodation divided by diopteric value of its refractive error
   D. range of accommodation multiplied by diopteric value of its refractive error

3. All of the following are the usual ocular features in this patient EXCEPT 3.______
   A. on wearing correction, the objects look smaller in size
   B. multitude of muscae volitantes
   C. there may be contraction of visual fields
   D. the subject may have angle closure glaucoma

4. All of the following are fundus features in this patient EXCEPT 4._______
   A. myopic crescent
   B. supertraction of the retina over the nasal side of the optic disc
   C. pseudopapillitis
   D. choroidal atrophy

5. The periphery of the retina may have which of the following changes in this patient? 5._______
   A. Snail track degeneration
   B. Lattice type of degeneration
   C. Lacquer cracks
   D. All of the above

6. The patient concerned is least likely to have 6._______
   A. hypertensive retinopathy
   B. diabetic retinopathy
   C. vascular obstruction
   D. all of the above

7. The nature of changes in retina and choroids in similar patients is 7._______
   A. degenerative
   B. inflammatory
   C. traumatic
   D. carcinomatous

8. Which change is expected to take place in vitreous in this patient? 8._______
   A. Vitreous synchysis
   B. Weiss reflex streak
   C. Hyaloid holes
   D. All of the above

Demographics: 15-year-old male
Chief complaint: Eye strain doing any kind of work near or distant, headache
Secondary complaints/symptoms: A point of light appears tailed off; sometimes dizziness, neurasthenia following studying
Patient's ocular history: Never used any spectacles before
Patient's medical history: Similar complaints for last four years
Medications taken by patient: nil
Patient's allergy history: nil
Family ocular history: nil
Family medical history: nil
Clinical findings: BCVA – OD –2.0 Dsph/+1.5 Dcyl x 180 – 6/5;
OS –2.5 Dsph/+1.0 Dcyl x 180 – 6/5
Pupils: OD and OS – NSNR
Hirshberg test: Orthophoria
Confrontation fields: Appear normal
Slit lamp: OD-OS – Anterior segment is normal
IOP: OD – 18 mmHg; OS – 18 mmHg
Fundus: OD-OS – C:D::0.3:1, foveal reflex normal

9. What is the diagnosis of the refractive error that this patient has? 9._______
   A. Myopia
   B. Hypermetropia
   C. Astigmatism
   D. Presbyopia

10. What type of lens would you prescribe for this patient? 10.______
    A. Lenticular
    B. Monofocal
    C. Bifocal
    D. Cylindrical

11. What is the name of the condition in which vertical curvature is less than the horizontal? 11.______
    A. Astigmatism with rule
    B. Direct astigmatism
    C. Inverse astigmatism
    D. Curvature astigmatism

12. Which technique is not useful in establishing the diagnosis of refractive error in this patient? 12.______
    A. Direct ophthalmoscope
    B. Streak retinoscope
    C. Priestly Smith retinoscope
    D. Stenopic slit

13. What cannot be the cause responsible for origin of this condition? 13.______
    A. Curvature
    B. Index
    C. Axial
    D. None of the above

14. Which of the following conditions causes irregular astigmatism? 14.______
    A. Incipient cataract
    B. Corneal ulcer
    C. Keratoconus
    D. All of the above

Demographics: 30-year-old female
Chief complaint: Deviation of right eye outward
Secondary complaints/symptoms: Strain when doing near work
Patient's ocular history: nil
Patient's medical history: Patient had fever and lower general health – 1 month
Medications taken by patient: Antipyretics
Patient's allergy history: nil
Family ocular history: nil
Family medical history: nil
Clinical findings: BCVA – OD 6/5, OS 6/5
Pupils: OD and OS – NSNR
Hirshberg test: RDS 15° → ADS 15°
Confrontation fields: Appear normal
Slit lamp: OD-OS – Anterior segment is normal
IOP: OD – 20 mmHg; OS – 20 mmHg
Fundus: OD-OS – C:D::0.3:1, foveal reflex normal

15. What is the most likely diagnosis of this condition? 15.______
    A. Concomitant convergent squint
    B. Concomitant divergent squint
    C. Paralytic convergent squint
    D. Paralytic divergent squint

16. What would the ocular movements be like in this patient? 16.______
    - A. Show no abnormality
    - B. Restricted in divergence
    - C. Restricted in convergence
    - D. Restricted in elevation and depression only

17. If this condition is allowed to persist for long without treatment, the likely outcome would be contracture of 17.______
    - A. lateral rectus
    - B. medial rectus
    - C. superior rectus
    - D. inferior rectus

18. What sensory adaptations are likely to take place in this patient in response to a situation where there is no treatment done? 18.______
    - A. Anomalous retinal correspondence
    - B. Amblyopia
    - C. Suppression
    - D. None of the above

19. What other factor is to be excluded in order to establish the diagnosis of divergence of the eyeball? 19.______
    - A. Asymmetry of orbits
    - B. Brachycephaly
    - C. Enophthalmos
    - D. All of the above

20. What is NOT useful in diagnosing this condition? 20.______
    - A. Prism bar cover test
    - B. Synoptophore
    - C. Indirect ophthalmoscopy
    - D. Hirshberg's test

21. What pattern would the patient observe on the Worth four-dot test? 21.______
    - A. Five dots
    - B. Two red dots only
    - C. Three dots only
    - D. None of the above

22. What grade of binocular vision would this patient be expected to have? 22.______
    - A. Simultaneous macular perception
    - B. Fusion
    - C. Stereopsis
    - D. All of the above

23. What is taken to be the normal amount of divergence? 23.______
    - A. 6-8 Δ
    - B. 1-2 Δ
    - C. 3-4 Δ
    - D. 4-6 Δ

24. What would be the nature of diplopia this patient would have if this squint was paralytic? 24.______
    - A. Crossed
    - B. Uncrossed
    - C. Sometimes crossed, sometimes uncrossed
    - D. No diplopia

25. Which corneal opacity is more deleterious to vision? 25.______
    A. Central nebular opacity
    B. Peripheral macular opacity
    C. Peripheral leucomatous opacity
    D. All are equally deleterious to vision

KEY (CORRECT ANSWERS)

1. A
2. A
3. D
4. C
5. D

6. D
7. A
8. D
9. C
10. D

11. C
12. A
13. C
14. D
15. B

16. A
17. A
18. D
19. D
20. C

21. D
22. D
23. A
24. A
25. A

EXAMINATION SECTION

TEST 1

DIRECTIONS: Use the patient information provided to answer the questions that follow. Each question or incomplete statement is followed by several suggested answers or completions. Select the one that BEST answers the question or completes the statement. *PRINT THE LETTER OF THE CORRECT ANSWER IN THE SPACE AT THE RIGHT.*

Demographics: 10-year-old male
Chief complaint: Strain on reading, difficulty in seeing blackboard
Secondary complaints/symptoms: Browache, heaviness of eyes
Patient's ocular history: nil
Patient's medical history: nil
Medications taken by patient: nil
Patient's allergy history: nil
Family ocular history: nil
Family medical history: nil
Clinical findings: BCVA – OD 6/12 → 6/5; OS 6/18 → 6/5 with pinhole
Pupils: OD and OS – NSNR
Hirschberg test: Orthophoria
Confrontation fields: Appear normal in both eyes
Slit lamp: Anterior segment is normal
IOP: OD – 16 mmHg; OS – 16 mmHg
Fundus: C:D::0.3:1, foveal reflex normal in both eyes

1. What is the probable cause of this condition? 1.______
    A. Refractive error
    B. Amblyopia
    C. Strabismus
    D. Anomalous retinal correspondence

2. What method of refraction would you prescribe for this patient? 2.______
    A. Dry retinoscopy B. Wet retinoscopy
    C. Direct ophthalmoscopy D. Indirect ophthalmoscopy

3. Which cycloplegic would you prefer to use in this age group? 3.______
    A. Atropine 1% B. Cyclopentolate 1%
    C. Tropicamide 1% D. Phenylepherine

4. What are the common side effects of cyclopentolate? 4.______
    A. Constipation and hallucination
    B. Hallucination and dry mouth
    C. Dry mouth and fever
    D. Constipation and fever

5. Cycloplegic refraction is indicated in all of the following EXCEPT 5.______
   A. young subjects B. fluctuating acuity
   C. high myopes D. glaucoma

6. What is not true of duchrome test? 6.______
   A. The test is based on chromatic aberration
   B. The red light is focused behind green light
   C. When the eye is fogged with plus spheres, the letter on red side should appear clearer
   D. If letter on the green side appears clearer, more minus correction is indicated

7. Which is not a test for subjective determination of refractive error for spherical power? 7.______
   A. Jackson cross cylinder B. Fogging
   C. Pinhole D. Stenopic slit

8. Which is not a test for subjective determination of refractive error for cylindrical power? 8.______
   A. Astigmatic dial B. Jackson cross cylinders
   C. Duchrome test D. Stenopic slit

9. All of the following points are to be kept in consideration while prescribing spectacles to this patient EXCEPT 9.______
   A. vertex distance of the trial lens should be measured
   B. the lens of the spectacles should have its focal point located at the far point of the eye
   C. low refraction index materials should be used in high myopia
   D. bilateral high myopes should be preferably given contact lenses

10. All of the following are true of refractive glasses in diabetics EXCEPT 10.______
   A. there is shift toward hyperopia
   B. refractive error fluctuates in diabetics
   C. the cause of fluctuation in diabetics is lens shape
   D. the refraction should be confirmed when glucose level is stable

11. Perceived images in a myopic are minified due to 11.______
   A. use of concave lens
   B. stretched apart spacing of photoreceptors
   C. both the use of concave lens and stretched apart spacing of photoreceptors
   D. none of the above

12. What refractive error does night (diurnal variation) introduce in the eye? 12.______
   A. Myopia B. Hyperopia
   C. Astigmatism D. Restricted field of vision

13. What formula gives the spherocylindrical transformation? 13.______
    A. x + y (axis z) becomes (x + y) – y (axis 90 degrees away from z)
    B. x + y (axis z) becomes (x – y) – y (axis 90 degrees away from z)
    C. x + y (axis z) becomes (x + y) – y (axis 180 degrees away from z)
    D. None of the above

14. What kid of spectacle prescription would you give if the astigmatism is different for near and far refraction? 14.______
    A. Separate reading glasses with astigmatism correction and separate distance glasses with astigmatic correction incorporated
    B. Bifocal glasses with different cylindrical correction for distance and near
    C. Only distance spectacles with astigmatic correction and near glasses left without astigmatic correction
    D. Only near spectacles with astigmatic correction and distance glasses left without astigmatic correction

15. Which of the following statements is NOT true? 15.______
    A. Minus lenses bring more peripheral field into view
    B. Plus lenses leave a peripheral scotoma between what is viewed through the lens and what is viewed looking around the lens
    C. Minus lens make straight lines viewed through the periphery of the lens appear concave with respect to the optical center of the lens
    D. Plus lens give pin-cushion distortion

16. What measures can be adopted to reduce the visual inconvenience caused by the spectacle correction of astigmatism? 16.______
    A. Rear surface grinding of cylinder
    B. Use of small diameter lenses
    C. Use of contact lens
    D. All of the above

4 (#1)

Demographics: 45-year-old male
Chief complaint: Difficulty reading newspaper and working on computer
Secondary complaints/symptoms: Dryness in both eyes
Patient's ocular history: nil
Patient's medical history: nil
Medications taken by patient: nil
Patient's allergy history: nil
Family ocular history: nil
Family medical history: nil
Clinical findings: BCVA – OD 6/12 corrected with +2.0 Dsph → 6/5; OS 6/18 corrected with +2.0 Dsph → 6/5; Add +1.0 Dsph both eyes for N 6
Pupils: NSNR
Hirschberg test: Orthophoria
Confrontation fields: Appear normal in both eyes
Slit lamp: Anterior segment is normal
IOP: 16 mmHg in both eyes
Fundus: C:D::0.3:1, foveal reflex normal in both eyes

17. Which glasses would you prefer for this patient? 17.______
    A. Near glasses
    B. Distance glasses
    C. Multifocal glasses
    D. Bifocal glasses

18. What are the characteristics of LASIK that you would do for a hyperopic patient? 18.______
    A. Excimer laser should deliver peripheral laser pulses to flatten peripheral cornea and steepen central cornea
    B. Large diameter flaps have to be used
    C. Several excimer lasers are capable of adequately correcting hyperopia with or without astigmatism up to a spherical equivalent of approximately +5D
    D. All of the above

19. Which of the following statements is not true for presbyopic LASIK? 19.______
    A. In monovision LASIK, dominant eye is corrected for distance viewing and other eye is corrected for near viewing
    B. Other procedure can be to reshape the central 3 mm zone so that it becomes multifocal but leave the most peripheral area of the cornea unchanged for intermediate and distance vision
    C. Centration is critical to avoid induced astigmatism
    D. Monovision LASIK does not cause any decrease in depth perception

20. What type of material can you use to make the spectacles to prevent aberrations if the refractive error is very high in this patient? 20.______
    A. Flint glass
    B. Plastic glasses
    C. Unleaded flint glass
    D. All of the above

21. What is the expected correcting lens that should be prescribed in a person who is aphakic? 21.______
    A. +10.0 Dsph / +3.0 Dcyl x 180°
    B. +10.0 Dsph / +3.0 x 90°
    C. +10.0 Dsph / -3.0 x 180°
    D. +10.0 Dsph / -3.0 x 90°

22. A spherocylindrical lens has all of the following characteristics EXCEPT 22.______
    A. greatest refractive power in one meridian and least refractive power perpendicular to that meridian
    B. spherical equivalent of a spherocylindrical lens can be calculated as equal to sphere plus (cylinder / 2)
    C. focuses a pencil of rays to a point
    D. circle of least confusion of the conoid of strum is located at the focal point of the spherical equivalent lens, whose power is midway between the diopteric power of the two cylindrical lenses that make up the astigmatic lens

23. What types of magnification will a correcting convex lens cause in this patient? 23.______
    A. Linear
    B. Axial
    C. Angular
    D. All of the above

24. The advantage of plastic lenses in spectacles instead of glass lenses is 24.______
    A. no danger of splintering
    B. more resistance to pitting
    C. fogging is not as quick as in glass
    D. all of the above

25. At what distance (in mm) should the correcting lens be held in front of the cornea in this patient? 25.______
    A. 15.7
    B. 14.0
    C. 12.3
    D. 10.5

KEY (CORRECT ANSWERS)

1. A	11. C	21. A
2. B	12. A	22. C
3. C	13. A	23. D
4. A	14. A	24. D
5. D	15. C	25. A
6. D	16. D	
7. D	17. C	
8. C	18. D	
9. C	19. D	
10. A	20. D	

TEST 2

DIRECTIONS: Use the patient information provided to answer the questions that follow. Each question or incomplete statement is followed by several suggested answers or completions. Select the one that BEST answers the question or completes the statement. *PRINT THE LETTER OF THE CORRECT ANSWER IN THE SPACE AT THE RIGHT.*

Demographics: 45-year-old male
Chief complaint: Difficulty reading newspaper and working on computer
Secondary complaints/symptoms: Dryness in both eyes
Patient's ocular history: nil
Patient's medical history: nil
Medications taken by patient: nil
Patient's allergy history: nil
Family ocular history: nil
Family medical history: nil
Clinical findings: BCVA – OD 6/12 corrected with +2.0 Dsph → 6/5; OS 6/18 corrected with +2.0 Dsph → 6/5; Add +1.0 Dsph both eyes for N 6
Pupils: NSNR
Hirschberg test: Orthophoria
Confrontation fields: Appear normal in both eyes
Slit lamp: Anterior segment is normal
IOP: 16 mmHg in both eyes
Fundus: C:D::0.3:1, foveal reflex normal in both eyes

1. How is correcting the refractive error with use of contact lens different from that with use of spectacles? 1.______
   A. The contact lens is closer to the anterior nodal point of the eye
   B. The contact lens is separated from eye with liquid medium rather than air
   C. The correction of myopia with contact lens results in larger retinal images than that created by spectacles
   D. All of the above

2. What type of contact lens could be used in this patient? 2.______
   A. Multifocal soft
   B. Multifocal rigid
   C. Bifocal soft
   D. Bifocal rigid

3. If the person is aphakic in one eye and correcting glasses are to be given for this eye, and the other eye is ametropic, what options for refractive correction would you prefer in this patient? 3.______
   I. Contact lens, if the ametropic eye is myopic
   II. Spectacle lens, if the ametropic eye is hyperopic
   III. Overcorrecting the optimal distance power of the aphakic contact lens and neutralizing this effect by prescribing an appropriate minus spectacle lens if the ametropic eye is myopic

   A. I only
   B. I and III only
   C. Either I, II or III
   C. None of the options

4. Regarding near work by myopic patient, which statement is correct? 4.______
   A. Do not use contact lens as accommodative requirement increases with their use
   B. Slide the high minus spectacles forward and increase their vertex distance, thus reducing the accommodative needs
   C. Remove the high minus spectacle lenses to get extra magnification needed for close fine work
   D. All of the above

5. Which is not true of the bifocal contact lens if used in this patient? 5.______
   A. Comfort may be compromised by the tendency of these lenses to position low
   B. It would be more successful in this patient than it would be in a patient who was myopic
   C. Proper orientation of segment bifocal designs is achieved by prism ballasting
   D. Lens truncation is of no help for proper orientation of segment bifocal spectacles

6. The contact lenses that can be prescribed for this patient are 6.______
   A. single vision contact lenses with glasses
   B. monovision lenses
   C. concentric lenses for simultaneous vision
   D. all of the above

7. Aspheric contact lenses have all of the following properties EXCEPT they 7.______
   A. are bifocal
   B. are progressive addition contact lenses
   C. provide simultaneous vision
   D. are thin lenses

8. Which of the following is not true regarding diffractive lenses? 8.______
   A. They are not easy to fit
   B. Rotational stability is not required
   C. Vision is not highly affected by pupil size
   D. A large range of powers is available in distance and near

Demographics: 15-year-old male
Chief complaint: Difficulty in seeing distant objects
Secondary complaints/symptoms: Recurring redness, itching in both eyes
Patient's ocular history: nil
Patient's medical history: nil
Medications taken by patient: nil
Patient's allergy history: nil
Family ocular history: Father had glasses to see distant objects
Family medical history: nil
Clinical findings: BCVA – OD 6/12 corrected with -3.0 Dsph → 6/5; OS 6/18 corrected with -4.0 Dsph → 6/5
Pupils: NSNR
Hirschberg test: Orthophoria
Confrontation fields: Appear normal in both eyes
Slit lamp: Anterior segment is normal
IOP: OD – 16 mmHg; OS – 18 mmHg
Fundus: C:D::0.3:1, foveal reflex normal in both eyes

9. The correcting glasses for this patient would lead to minification of retinal image due to 9.______
   A. reverse Galilean telescopic effect
   B. stretched apart spacing of photoreceptors
   C. both of the above
   D. neither A nor B

10. Which is not true of the refractive correction that this patient should be given? 10.______
    A. Constant wearing of spectacles should be advised
    B. Even for near work, the use of glasses in earlier stages is important
    C. A full correction should not be ordered; the refractive error should be under-corrected
    D. In very high myopes, contact lens should be prescribed

11. Which of the following is not true of LASIK used for correction of myopia? 11.______
    A. Customized LASIK is useful for correction of defects like comma, spherical or trefoil
    B. The ocular aberration is measured with aberrometer
    C. Astigmatism up to 5 D can be corrected
    D. LASIK corrects some of the retinal lesions in myopia

12. Which of the following surgeries can be useful for correction of this patient's refractive error? 12.______
    A. Radial keratotomy
    B. LASIK
    C. Synthetic intra-corneal inlays
    D. All of the above

13. Which of the following is not a contraindication for performance of LASIK in this patient? 13.______
    A. Ectatic corneal disease
    B. Dry eyes
    C. Previously operated dacryocystorhinostomy
    D. Glaucoma

14. What test should you perform before taking the patient for LASIK? 14.______
    A. Keratometry
    B. Corneal topography
    C. Ultrasound pachymetry
    D. All of the above

15. Which statement is not true regarding LASIK done for myopia? 15.______
    A. Tonometry must be done before cutting flap
    B. The flap cut includes epithelium and a thin part of Bowman's membrane
    C. The flap has to be cut when surface is wet
    D. The ablation has to be done when surface is dry

16. Which is NOT a microkeratome-related complication of LASIK surgery? 16.______
    A. Corneal perforation
    B. Incomplete flap
    C. Thin flap
    D. Flap wrinkling

17. Which is NOT an optical complication of LASIK? 17.______
    A. Central islands
    B. Diffuse lamellar keratitis
    C. Bleeding from limbal vessels
    D. Interface haze

18. A posterior segment change that LASIK can bring about is 18.______
    A. retinal detachment
    B. reduced retinal nerve fiber layer thickness
    C. optic neuropathy
    D. all of the above

19. What precautions should be observed in a patient in whom LASIK is done after penetrating keratoplasty? 19.______
    I. LASIK should be done at least 18 months to two years after primary surgery
    II. LASIK should be done after all sutures of PK have been removed
    III. A 180 micron depth plate is mandatory in such eyes

    A. I and II
    B. II and III
    C. I, II and III
    D. None

20. Which of the following is not true of regression seen after LASIK surgery? 20.______
    A. The rate of regression is higher if the myopia is high
    B. Maximal regression usually occurs between 2-4 weeks but can be seen up to six months after surgery
    C. Proliferation of keratocytes with a remodulation of the corneal stroma causes regression
    D. Reactive epithelial hyperplasia is not responsible for regression

21. Which is true of precautions to be observed if the repeat LASIK surgery is done in a patient? 21.______
    I. Thinner depth plate should be used if more than six months have elapsed since first LASIK surgery
    II. If repeat surgery is done, it should be done after post-operative refraction is stable over four weeks
    III. Any corneal ectasia is a contraindication of LASIK surgery

    A. I and II B. I, II and III C. II and III D. I and III

22. The advantages of LASIK over PRK do NOT include 22.______
    A. minimal need for steroids
    B. reduced incidence of corneal haze, regression and scarring
    C. healing takes more time and depends on the diameter of the flap
    D. the correction achieved is more predictable

Demographics: 20-year-old female
Chief complaint: Difficulty in reading from blackboard; headache and giddiness following studies for long intervals
Secondary complaints/symptoms: nil
Patient's ocular history: Similar complaints over the past year
Patient's medical history: nil
Medications taken by patient: nil
Patient's allergy history: nil
Family ocular history: Father had glasses to see distant objects
Family medical history: nil
Clinical findings: BCVA – OD 6/18 corrected with -3.0 Dsph / -1.5 Dcyl x 90° → 6/5; OS 6/18 corrected with –3.5 Dsph / -1.75 Dcyl x 90° → 6/5
Pupils: NSNR
Hirschberg test: Orthophoria
Confrontation fields: Appear normal in both eyes
Slit lamp: Anterior segment is normal
IOP: OD – 16 mmHg; OS – 16 mmHg
Fundus: C:D::0.3:1, foveal reflex normal in both eyes

23. What type of contact lenses can be used to correct astigmatism? 23.______
    A. Spherical soft
    B. Toric RGP
    C. Spherical RGP
    D. All of the above

24. The sphero-cylindrical lenses CANNOT correct _________ astigmatism. 24.______
    A. irregular
    B. with-the-rule
    C. against-the-rule
    D. oblique

25. What is not true of LASIK done following radial keratotomy in an eye that is left with residual refractive error?
    A. LASIK should be done in an eye with radial keratotomy done but having eight or fewer incisions
    B. In this LASIK one should create smaller and thinner flaps than usual
    C. LASIK should not be done if RK surgery was complicated by micro-macro-perforations
    D. LASIK should not be done if there are epithelial plugs present in the incision

---

KEY (CORRECT ANSWERS)

1. D	11. D	21. C
2. B	12. D	22. C
3. C	13. C	23. C
4. D	14. D	24. A
5. D	15. B	25. B
6. D	16. D	
7. A	17. C	
8. A	18. D	
9. C	19. C	
10. C	20. D	

TEST 3

DIRECTIONS: Use the patient information provided to answer the questions that follow. Each question or incomplete statement is followed by several suggested answers or completions. Select the one that BEST answers the question or completes the statement. *PRINT THE LETTER OF THE CORRECT ANSWER IN THE SPACE AT THE RIGHT.*

Demographics: 20-year-old female
Chief complaint: Difficulty in reading from blackboard; headache and giddiness following studies for long intervals
Secondary complaints/symptoms: nil
Patient's ocular history: Similar complaints over the past year
Patient's medical history: nil
Medications taken by patient: nil
Patient's allergy history: nil
Family ocular history: Father had glasses to see distant objects
Family medical history: nil
Clinical findings: BCVA – OD 6/18 corrected with -3.0 Dsph / -1.5 Dcyl x 90° → 6/5; OS 6/18 corrected with –3.5 Dsph / -1.75 Dcyl x 90° → 6/5
Pupils: NSNR
Hirschberg test: Orthophoria
Confrontation fields: Appear normal in both eyes
Slit lamp: Anterior segment is normal
IOP: OD – 16 mmHg; OS – 16 mmHg
Fundus: C:D::0.3:1, foveal reflex normal in both eyes

1. Which is NOT true of residual astigmatism? 1.______
   A. It is the astigmatism that remains after correction of corneal astigmatism
   B. It can be caused by a toric crystalline lens
   C. It can be caused by a warped contact lens
   D. Residual astigmatism cannot be caused by a toric back surface on the cornea

2. Which is NOT true of the correction of astigmatism with contact lens? 2.______
   A. Spherical soft lenses can correct total astigmatism (up to 1D) if it is not more than 1/3 of the spherical correction
   B. If astigmatism is greater than 1D, then rigid lens or a toric soft lens would be needed
   C. When spherical soft lenses are used to mask astigmatism, thinner lenses are preferred over standard thickness lenses
   D. None of the above

3. Toric soft contact lenses are contraindicated in 3.______
   A. irregular corneal astigmatism
   B. patients with lid closure abnormality
   C. Bell's palsy
   D. all of the above

4. Which is NOT true for the steps checked during fitting of a toric soft lens? 4.______
   A. A base curve is selected by converting the mean of K reading to millimeter and add 0.7 mm
   B. An over-refraction has to be done
   C. The aim is that no movement of lens should be seen while blinking
   D. Keratometry mires and retinoscopy reflexes should be sharp

5. Which is true for double slab off lenses? 5.______
   I. Base curve is selected by subtracting 4D from the flattest K reading
   II. These lenses are suggested for patients with 1 to 2D of astigmatism
   III. They work poorly for those with oblique astigmatism
   IV. Tight lids or small palpebral fissure are contraindications to double slab off lenses

   A. I, II and III B. II, III and IV C. I, III and IV D. I, II, III, IV

6. What method is used to check the rotation of soft toric contact lens? 6.______
   A. By etch or laser mark at 3 o'clock and 9 o'clock position
   B. By using a trial frame that is aligned with lens marking
   C. Slit lamp with a reticule that can be lined up with lens marking
   D. All of the above

7. Which is NOT true for the orientation of the toric soft contact lens? 7.______
   A. When placed on the eye, if the lens rotates in a clockwise direction, the amount of deviation in degrees is added to the spectacle axis and vice versa
   B. Toric soft lens should be fit slightly loose if possible
   C. When the lens assumes its final position, rotation on blinking should be less than 5°
   D. Movement in the same direction on successive blinks indicates a tight fit

8. Which of the following statements is NOT true of toric soft contact lens? 8.______
   A. Discomfort due to contact lens may be related to excess movement
   B. Poor vision with contact lens may be caused by inability of the lens to stabilize properly
   C. In oblique astigmatism, orientation is easy to achieve
   D. Edge lift off is a sign of a potential bad fit of contact lens

9. Which of the following statements is false? 9.______
   A. A patient with 1D of astigmatism should be given spherical soft contact lenses if total astigmatism is not more than 1/3 of spherical correction
   B. Astigmatism of more than 1D (up to 2D) can be corrected by spherical RGP lens
   C. Astigmatism of more than 2D will require toric RGP lens
   D. None of the above

10. Which is a characteristic of astigmatic keratotomy? 10.______
   A. It is useful for correcting astigmatism of approximately 3D or higher
   B. An arch-shaped deep incision (approximately 80% of thickness of cornea) is placed in the axis of strongest curvature in the periphery of cornea
   C. Perforation of eye may occur from the incision
   D. All of the above

Demographics: 15-year-old female
Chief complaints: Diminution of vision in both eyes R/E > L/E; inability to gain good vision with previous spectacles prescription given one month ago
Secondary complaints: A cone-like projection in cornea of right eye; L/E cornea appears normal
Patient's ocular history: Nil
Patient's medical history: Nil
Medications taken by patient: Nil
Patient's allergic history: Nil
Family ocular history: Father and brother had high myopia
Family medical history: Nil
Clinical Findings: BCVA – OD 6/18 corrected to 6/9 with glasses; OS 6/12 corrected to 6/9 with glasses; on retinoscopy, confusing retinoscopic pattern with 'scissors' movement
Pupils: NSNR
Confrontation fields: Appear normal in both eyes
Slit lamp examination: Cone-like projection in center of right eye; no such cone-like projection is clearly visible in left eye
IOP: Not possible to record with Goldman applanation tonometer
Fundus: C:D::0.3:1, Foveal reflex – normal in both eyes.

11. Corneal topography is used for assessing the type of contact lens to be fitted for this patient. What is not true of corneal topography? 11.______
   A. Color-coded topographic map of the cornea is made
   B. Blue and green colors represent flat areas
   C. Yellow, orange and red are warm colors
   D. The symmetric bow-tie configuration is an uncommon topographic pattern

12. Which of the following are true of the disinfection of soft contact lenses? 12.______
    I. The rubbing of lenses with the finger is as important as the surfactant cleaner in removing material from lens
    II. Lenses treated with heat rather than chemical disinfection tend to develop deposits more quickly because heat denatures the deposit protein
    III. Use surfactant cleaner before enzyme treatment

    A. I, II and III B. II and III C. I and II D. I and III

13. Which of the following is NOT a treatment of keratoconus? 13.______
    A. Lamellar keratoplasty
    B. Penetrating keratoplasty
    C. Rigid gas permeable lens
    D. Intraocular lens

14. What diseases would jeopardize the success of keratoplasty – lamellar or penetrating – if present in this patient? 14.______
    I. Herpes simplex keratitis
    II. Herpes zoster ophthalmicus
    III. Stevens Johnson syndrome
    IV. Dacryocystitis

    A. I, II and III B. II, III and IV C. I, III and IV D. I, II, III and IV

15. Which is not an indication for cessation of treatment with contact lens and preference for keratoplasty? 15.______
    A. It is indicated in patients who can no longer be successfully fit with contact lenses
    B. It is indicated in patients in whom corneal scarring precludes good vision
    C. It is indicated in patients with perforation of cornea
    D. It is indicated in patients in whom corrective spectacles are not effective in treating the patient

16. Which is NOT true of contact lenses regarding treatment of keratoconus? 16.______
    A. Except for vision correction, wearing contact lenses medically benefits the keratoconic eye
    B. Contact lens fitting in keratoconic eye is difficult and time consuming
    C. Quality of vision correction is often suboptimal
    D. The visual benefit of wearing contact lens is the result of their ability to neutralize optically the irregular and distorted anterior corneal surface

17. Among the investigations to be done before taking a patient of corneal opacity for penetrating keratoplasty is 17.______
    A. laser interferometry
    B. confocal microscopy
    C. gonioscopy
    D. all of the above

18. Which of the following are diseases that are contraindicated for the use of donor tissue for penetrating keratoplasty? 18.______

I. Congenital rubella II. Reye's syndrome
III. Rabies IV. Hepatitis B surface antigen

A. I, II and III B. II, III and IV C. I, II and III D. I, II, III, IV

19. Which of the following factors does not have an influence on survival of corneal transplant? 19.______

A. Age of donor
B. Presence of retinoblastoma in eye of donor
C. Endothelial cell density of the donor cornea
D. Prior intraocular surgery in donor's eye

20. Which of the following is not a problem associated with the donation of an infant's eye cornea for transplantation? 20.______

A. The thin infant cornea is likely to fold upon itself during handling
B. There is myopic shift after keratoplasty with infant donor cornea
C. The infant's cornea gets rejected more easily than an adult cornea
D. Small diameter of cornea creates problem during eye donation surgery

21. Which of the following is not a method to evaluate endothelium? 21.______

A. Specular microscopy
B. Indirect illumination by slit lamp
C. Phase contrast microscopy
D. Transmitted light microscopy

22. All of the following are conditions to be satisfied before performing penetrating keratoplasty in this patient EXCEPT 22.______

A. intraocular pressure should be reduced
B. an attempt should be made to increase corneal neovascularisation with use of preoperative steroids to accelerate healing of the donor-host interface
C. pupil should be constricted in the recipient
D. a videokeratography should be used to rule out previous PRK or LASIK in the donor

23. What complications is this patient likely to have during trephination of her cornea for doing keratoplasty even when adequate preoperative preparation of eye has been done? 23.______

A. Scleral collapse
B. Sudden increase in intraocular pressure
C. Retinal detachment
D. None of the above

24. What is not true of keratoconus? 24.______
    A. The apex of the cone is usually oriented downwards and towards the nose
    B. The cone is thinner than the rest of cornea
    C. Increasing myopia and progressive irregular astigmatism are characteristics of the condition
    D. Similar to the cone in center, the peripheral cornea is also much thinner than normal cornea

25. Which are true of progression of keratoconus? 25.______
    I. Keratoconus usually begins during the teen years
    II. Keratoconus tends to have periods of cone progression interspersed with periods of corneal stability until middle age
    III. At some point between 35 and 45 years, keratoconus cornea usually stabilizes and no further change will be seen

    A. I and II B. II and III C. I and III D. I, II, III

KEY (CORRECT ANSWERS)

1. D	11. D	21. B
2. C	12. A	22. B
3. D	13. D	23. A
4. C	14. D	24. D
5. D	15. D	25. D
6. D	16. A	
7. B	17. D	
8. C	18. D	
9. D	19. A	
10. D	20. C	

TEST 4

DIRECTIONS: Use the patient information provided to answer the questions that follow. Each question or incomplete statement is followed by several suggested answers or completions. Select the one that BEST answers the question or completes the statement. *PRINT THE LETTER OF THE CORRECT ANSWER IN THE SPACE AT THE RIGHT.*

1. In patients with advanced keratoconus with high myopia (-20 D to –25 D) the option for fitting contact lens is 1.______
   A. thin RGP lens design
   B. the piggyback technique (a rigid lens riding on a soft lens)
   C. RGP semiscleral lens design
   D. all of the above

Demographics: 50-year-old male
Chief complaint: Pain, redness and diminution of vision four weeks after cataract surgery with IOL implantation in right eye
Secondary complaint: Headache
Medications taken by the patient: Topical and systemic antibiotics, systemic analgesics
Patient's ocular history: Had diminution of vision in both eyes
Patient's medical history: Nil
Family ocular history: Nil
Family medical history: Nil
Examination: BCVA – OD HMCF, projection of rays accurate; OS 6/60
Pupils: OD – Sluggish reaction to light; OS – NSNR
Confrontation fields: Appear normal in both eyes
Slit lamp examination: OD – Hypopyon positive, conjunctival congestion, circumcorneal congestion; OS – White reflex in pupillary area
IOP: OD – 22 mmHg; OS – 18 mmHg
Fundus: OD – Glow is dull; OS – C:D::0.3:1, foveal reflex normal

2. What would be the preferred mode of treatment in this patient at this instance? 2.______
   A. Intravenous antibiotics and topical antibiotics
   B. Immediate vitrectomy
   C. Intensive systemic antibiotic therapy
   D. Systemic and topical steroids and topical antibiotics

3. Which is NOT an indication of vitrectomy? 3.______
   A. Post-operative endophthalmitis with light perception only
   B. Endophthalmitis with retained intraocular foreign body
   C. Sterile endophthalmitis
   D. Fungal endophthalmitis

4. What dosage of intraviteal antibiotic must be given at the end of vitrectomy? 4.______
   A. Same dose as usually given
   B. Double the usual dose
   C. Half the usual dose
   D. 1/10 of the usual intravitreal dose of antibiotics

5. Which is a condition that precludes use of intravitreal antibiotic in a patient? 5.______
   A. Retinal detachment B. Open angle glaucoma
   C. Perception of light negative D. All of the above

6. What are the indications of vitrectomy in a patient with endophthalmitis? 6.______
   I. Fungal endophthalmitis
   II. No relief following two intravitreal injections
   III. Delayed vitrectomy even when infection controlled but multiple vitreous opacities which hamper vision

   A. I and II B. II and III C. I, II and III D. I and III

7. What is not the site of intravitreal injection in an eye? 7.______
   A. 3 mm from limbus in aphakic eyes
   B. 5 mm from limbus in eyes with anterior retinal detachment
   C. 3.5 mm from limbus in pseudophakic eyes
   D. 4 mm from limbus in phakic eye

8. What should not be done in an intravitreal injection? 8.______
   A. Prior to intravitreal injection, do ultrasound to rule out retinal detachment
   B. Bevel of needle should face posterior
   C. Check of intraocular pressure of the eye
   D. 21g needle used to aspirate 0.2 ml vitreous

9. What should be the volume of total dose of an intravitreal injection? 9.______
   A. 0.2 ml B. 0.3 ml C. 0.1 ml D. 0.4 ml

10. Which statement is true of drugs used for intravitreal injection? 10.______
   A. Combination of vancomycin and ceftazidime is ideal in view of the multiplicity of organisms
   B. Fluconazole is used for intravitreal injection in fungal endophthalmitis
   C. Intravitreal aminoglycosides can cause macular toxicity
   D. All of the above

11. The intravitreal injection dose of dexamethasone is 11.______
   A. 400 μg B. 200 μg C. 300 μg D. 100 μg

12. The advantages of vitrectomy include all of the following EXCEPT 12.______
    A. vitrectomy allows reduction of bulk organisms
    B. greater access of antibiotics to the ocular tissue
    C. specimen for microbiological studies is obtained as part of vitrectomy procedure
    D. vitrectomy cures endophthalmitis even when the effective antibiotics are not administered

13. What is not true for the vitrectomy done in an eye with endophthalmitis? 13.______
    A. Core vitrectomy is done
    B. Low cutting and high suction rate is utilized
    C. Presence of choroidal detachment can make proper placement of infusion cannula difficult
    D. Surface retinal exudates are left behind

14. Which is an indication for removal of IOL in management of pseudophakic endophthalmitis? 14.______
    A. Fungal endophthalmitis
    B. Propionibacterium acne endophthalmitis
    C. Poor visualization due to intraocular lens related opacities
    D. All of the above

15. Which of the following are true for evisceration done in endophthalmitis? 15.______
    I. Done if patient presents with loss of perception of light
    II. Done if signs of early pan-ophthalmitis are present
    III. Artificial eye is placed in socket soon after evisceration is done

    A. I and II B. II and III C. I and III D. I, II and III

16. Which is NOT an ocular complication following vitrectomy in endophthalmitis? 16.______
    A. Cataract
    B. Rhegmatogenous retinal detachment
    C. Macular infarction
    D. Tendency for sclerotomies to enlarge

17. The advantages of Povidone iodine for skin preparation in prevention of post-surgical endophthalmitis include all of the following EXCEPT 17.______
    A. minimally toxic
    B. even solution as dilute as 1 % is effective
    C. has a broad spectrum of activity
    D. inexpensive

18. The most common cause of chronic endophthalmitis is 18.______
    A. propionibacterium acne B. staphylococcus epidermidis
    C. corynebacterium D. fungi

19. All of the following are true of bleb-associated endophthalmitis EXCEPT 19.______
    A. in most cases of late bleb associated endophthalmitis, the Siedel's test is negative
    B. bleb associated endophthalmitis is same as blebitis
    C. streptococcus species is most commonly implicated
    D. this risk is higher in eyes with thin walled cystic blebs

20. Which is NOT true of the samples to be used for culture studies in diagnosis of a patient with endophthalmitis? 20.______
    A. Vitreous samples are most important
    B. Aqueous samples are often negative despite positive vitreous culture
    C. Anterior chamber culture should not be performed in all cases
    D. A negative vitreous culture may be accompanied by a positive anterior chamber culture

Demographics: 15-year-old male
Chief complaint: Trauma in right eye with a cricket ball, periorbital swelling and redness is positive
Secondary complaint: Difficulty in moving right eyeball upwards
Medications taken by the patient: Systemic antibiotics and systemic analgesics
Patient's ocular history: Had diminution of vision in both eyes
Patient's medical history: Nil
Family ocular history: Nil
Family medical history: Nil
Examination: BCVA – OD 6/9; OS 6/5; enophthalmos in right eye
Pupils: OD – NSNR; OS – NSNR
Confrontation fields: Appear normal in both eyes
Slit lamp examination: OD – mild conjunctival congestion, anterior segment is normal; OS – anterior segment is normal
IOP: OD – 18 mmHg; OS – 18 mmHg
Fundus: OD – C:D::0.3:1, foveal reflex normal; OS – C:D::0.3:1, foveal reflex normal

21. What will be the investigation of choice that should be performed for this patient? 21.______
    A. X-ray orbit
    B. MRI scan head and orbit
    C. Urine-sugar and albumin
    D. Blood picture for TLC, DLC, ESR

22. Which statement about the role of ultrasound in orbital trauma is false? 22.______
    A. Ultrasound can show scleral rupture
    B. It has a role only in cases of blunt trauma
    C. It helps in precise localization of foreign body
    D. Even the magnetic properties of foreign body can be determined

23. What should be the first line of treatment in this patient, along with giving systemic oral antibiotics and oral analgesics? 23.______
    A. Systemic steroids B. Intravenous antibiotics
    C. Topical antibiotics D. Topical steroids

24. What are the indications of surgical intervention in a blowout fracture of the orbit? 24.______
    A. Fracture floor of orbit when more than half of it is involved
    B. Diplopia after two weeks
    C. Positive forced duction test due to entrapment of muscles
    D. All of the above

25. Which is NOT true of a blowout fracture of roof of orbit? 25.______
    A. Incidence in children is 20 times less than in adults
    B. Indication of repair is roof bone displacement causing symptoms
    C. CSF leak into the orbit
    D. Blow-out fracture of roof is more common than blowout fracture of floor of orbit

---

KEY (CORRECT ANSWERS)

1. D	11. A	21. A
2. A	12. D	22. B
3. C	13. B	23. A
4. D	14. D	24. D
5. D	15. A	25. D
6. C	16. C	
7. B	17. B	
8. B	18. A	
9. A	19. B	
10. D	20. C	

TEST 5

DIRECTIONS: Use the patient information provided to answer the questions that follow. Each question or incomplete statement is followed by several suggested answers or completions. Select the one that BEST answers the question or completes the statement. *PRINT THE LETTER OF THE CORRECT ANSWER IN THE SPACE AT THE RIGHT.*

Demographics: 15-year-old male
Chief complaint: Trauma in right eye with a cricket ball, periorbital swelling and redness is positive
Secondary complaint: Difficulty in moving right eyeball upwards
Medications taken by the patient: Systemic antibiotics and systemic analgesics
Patient's ocular history: Had diminution of vision in both eyes
Patient's medical history: Nil
Family ocular history: Nil
Family medical history: Nil
Examination: BCVA – OD 6/9; OS 6/5; enophthalmos in right eye
Pupils: OD – NSNR; OS – NSNR
Confrontation fields: Appear normal in both eyes
Slit lamp examination: OD – mild conjunctival congestion, anterior segment is normal; OS – anterior segment is normal
IOP: OD – 18 mmHg; OS – 18 mmHg
Fundus: OD – C:D::0.3:1, foveal reflex normal; OS – C:D::0.3:1, foveal reflex normal

1. The properties of a blowout fracture include all of the following EXCEPT 1.______
    A. it is produced from injury with non-penetrating convex object of greater diameter than the orbital margin
    B. the tissue of orbit is compressed and increased pressure is transmitted to the wall of which the more delicate portions are fractured
    C. if the impact is big, even the orbital rim can be involved
    D. floor is the usual site of fracture, possibly because the weak area is convex in shape and bulges slightly upwards behind the eyeball

2. The most common site of a blowout fracture is the 2.______
    A. superior wall of orbit
    B. anterior part of orbital floor
    C. posterior part of orbital floor medial to the infraorbital groove and canal
    D. medial wall of orbit

3. The reason for high incidence of fracture at this site is the 3.______
   A. extreme thinness of the bone at this point
   B. close proximity of the upwardly inclined bone of the posterior orbital floor to the globe
   C. site of fracture lies directly beneath the geometrical orbital axis along which it is presumed the eyeball is pushed as a result of a direct frontal blow
   D. all of the above

4. The sign of medial orbital wall fracture may include all of the following EXCEPT 4.______
   A. bleeding from nose
   B. opacification of frontal sinus
   C. narrowing of palpebral fissure on attempted abduction
   D. retraction of globe

5. Which is true of enophthalmos associated with a blowout fracture? 5.______
   A. It is usually initially absent
   B. It develops in 10 days to two weeks
   C. The severity of enophthalmos may continue to increase for about six months
   D. All of the above

6. Which of the following statements is NOT true about blowout fractures of the inferior orbital wall? 6.______
   A. Downward gaze may be restricted due to pinched inferior rectus
   B. Upward gaze is not restricted
   C. Diplopia occurs in both up and down gaze
   D. Forced duction and differential intraocular pressure tests are positive

7. What is NOT true of orbital roof fractures? 7.______
   A. More common in young children than in adults
   B. They occur because children have softer bones
   C. They occur because children do not have frontal sinus pneumatization
   D. Chronic disturbance of vision, ocular motility and eyelid function after recovery from orbital roof fracture is common

8. Which of the following are true of superior orbital fissure syndrome? 8.______
   I. Cranial nerve III, IV and VI may be involved
   II. There may be upper eyelid ptosis and proptosis
   III. Sensation is lost in distribution of cranial nerve VI

   A. I and II   B. II and III   C. I and III   D. I, II and III

9. Which of the following are false regarding supraorbital-frontal fractures? 9.______
   I. Supraorbital-frontal area fractures may cause significant indirect optic nerve trauma with subsequent loss of vision from traumatic optic neuropathy
   II. Proptosis is accompanied by a downward displacement of globe
   III. Frontal lobe injury often accompanies frontal-supraorbital fracture

   A. I and II
   B. II and III
   C. I, II and III
   D. None of the above

10. All of the following are true of CT scan in detection of a foreign body EXCEPT 10.______
    A. can suggest intraorbital foreign body composition by radiodensity
    B. thin cuts < 1.5 mm are the best ones
    C. can detect fragments of wood
    D. can accurately locate IOFB, even multiple and anterior located ones

Demographics: 50-year-old female
Chief complaint: Diminution of vision in both eyes, left eye > right eye – one year
Secondary complaint: Recurrent itching and redness
Medications taken by the patient: Antidiabetics
Patient's ocular history: Recurrent itching and redness
Patient's medical history: Diabetes for 15 years
Family ocular history: Mother operated for cataract in both eyes
Family medical history: Mother was also diabetic
Examination: BCVA – OD 6/12 → 6/6P; OS 6/12 → 6/9
Pupils: OD – NSNR; OS – NSNR
Confrontation fields: Appear normal in both eyes
Slit lamp examination: OD and OS – anterior segment is normal
IOP: OD – 20 mmHg; OS – 20 mmHg
Fundus: OD and OS – C:D::0.3:1, foveal reflex dull, small dot hemorrhages in macular area, soft exudates in macular area
Fluorescein angiography: Leak in the macular region in both eyes

11. Which statement is NOT true of laser treatment in a patient with diabetic macular edema? 11.______
    A. In focal diabetic edema, do focal laser
    B. In diffuse diabetic macular edema, do macular grid laser
    C. If both types of edema, do both focal and grid laser
    D. If both macular edema and rest of the retinal involvement, panretinal photocoagulation is done first followed by macular laser

12. If there is cataract with background diabetic retinopathy in a patient, what should be done? 12.______

I. Do macular laser first followed by cataract surgery
II. Phacoemulsification is the surgery of choice
III. Do cataract surgery first followed by macular laser

A. I and II
B. II and III
C. I and III
D. None of the above

13. In what ways does cataract surgery not effect the course of diabetes? 13.______

A. Cataract surgery increases the risk of cystoid macular edema
B. Cataract surgery increases risk of progression of retinopathy
C. Cataract surgery increases risk of anterior segment neovascularisation
D. Cataract surgery increases risk of rhegmatogenous retinal detachment

14. Which is NOT true of the laser burns placed in treatment of panretinal photocoagulation? 14.______

A. Gray-white burns are produced
B. Topical anesthesia is sufficient
C. Treatment is more heavy superiorly than inferiorly
D. Confluent treatment is needed in neovascularisation elsewhere

15. Which of the following are true of scatter photocoagulation done for background diabetic retinopathy? 15.______

I. Laser burns are placed in mid-peripheral retina
II. Burns are placed at 500 μm from optic disc
III. It spares the papillomacular bundle
IV. It remains 1 DD from center of macula

A. I, II and III
B. II, III and IV
C. I, III and IV
D. I, II and IV

16. Which management strategy is not right from the following choices? 16.______

A. Mild NPDR (microaneurysms only) – Optimize medical treatment, and glucose, blood pressure and lipid control
B. Moderate NPDR – Optimize medical treatment, and glucose, blood pressure and lipid control
C. Severe NPDR – Laser photocoagulation, panretinal photocoagulation, optimize medical treatment
D. Proliferative diabetic retinopathy – Immediate vitrectomy

17. Which is not the treatment modality for treatment of macular edema? 17.______

A. Pars plana vitrectomy with removal of internal limiting membrane
B. Intravitreal injection of triamcinolone
C. Optical coherence tomography
D. Grid photocoagulation

18. Which is a side effect of laser treatment? 18.______
    A. Field constriction
    B. Nyctalopia
    C. Serous or choroidal detachment
    D. All of the above

19. The complications of laser treatment include all of the following EXCEPT 19.______
    A. foveal burns
    B. macular edema
    C. corneal burns
    D. ptosis

20. Which of the following is a risk factor for progression of NPDR to PDR? 20.______
    A. Flourescein leakage
    B. Capillary loss on FA
    C. Capillary dilatation on FA
    D. All of the above

21. Which is NOT true of the role of FA in a patient of diabetic retinopathy? 21.______
    A. FA of the macula in presence of CSME is fundamental for the detection of treatable lesions
    B. It is absolutely indicated to diagnose NVE and NVD
    C. FA is useful to show capillary non-perfusion areas
    D. Capillary dilatation on FA, fluorescein leakage and capillary loss on FA are all closely correlated with ETDRS colour fundus photographic retinopathy severity levels

22. The effects of diabetes on macula include all of the following EXCEPT 22.______
    A. macular edema
    B. total retinal detachment
    C. non-perfusion of parafoveal capillaries
    D. lamellar or full thickness retinal hole formation

23. Which statement is false? 23.______
    A. Diabetic women contemplating pregnancy should have a complete eye examination before conception
    B. Pregnant women with diabetes should have their eyes examined early in each trimester of pregnancy
    C. Diabetes retinopathy in the pregnant diabetic patients without evidence of retinopathy at beginning of pregnancy may also progress during pregnancy
    D. Patients with evidence of proliferative diabetic retinopathy should not undertake pregnancy

24. The high-risk characteristics demonstrated by DRS are 24.______
    A. moderate to severe NVD (greater than standard photograph 10A)
    B. any NVD with vitreous or pre-retinal hemorrhage
    C. moderate to severe NVE with vitreous or pre-retinal hemorrhage
    D. all of the above

25. Which is NOT true of the various risk factors associated with diabetes? 25.______
    A. Elevated glycosylated hemoglobin is associated with increased incidence of severe retinopathy
    B. Proteinuria is associated with increased incidence of severe retinopathy
    C. Myopia > 2 D is associated with increased incidence of severe retinopathy
    D. Severity of retinopathy is related to duration of diabetes

26. Which of the following is an indication to do laser PHC in patients having NPDR? 26.______
    A. Severe NPDR in both eyes
    B. Pregnant ladies with NPDR
    C. Diabetics likely to undergo cataract surgery
    D. All of the above

27. What remedy is NOT offered for a patient in whom the pupil does not dilate for laser? 27.______
    A. Control diabetes
    B. Use atropine
    C. Use laser pupilloplasty
    D. Do laser indirect ophthalmoscopy

28. Diabetic vitrectomy is not different from usual vitrectomies in which aspect? 28.______
    A. There is presence of posterior vitreous detachment
    B. Increased risk of intraoperative hemorrhage as multiple vascular epicenters
    C. Multiple instrumentation
    D. Increased risk of retinal break formation

29. What change in the retina is NOT expected following laser treatment of diabetic retinopathy? 29.______
    A. Reduced caliber of vessels
    B. Angry look of NVE/NVD lost
    C. Fibrous component disappears
    D. Decrease in number of hemorrhages and exudates

30. Which of the following is not true of grid laser treatment of diabetic retinopathy? 30.______
    A. Done for focal macular edema
    B. Done for diffuse diabetic macular edema
    C. Done for ischemic maculopathy
    D. In grid laser, burns should be moderate and not chalky white

KEY (CORRECT ANSWERS)

1. C	11. D	21. B
2. D	12. A	22. B
3. D	13. D	23. C
4. B	14. C	24. D
5. D	15. A	25. C
6. B	16. D	26. D
7. D	17. C	27. A
8. D	18. D	28. A
9. D	19. D	29. C
10. C	20. D	30. A

EXAMINATION SECTION

TEST 1

DIRECTIONS: Use the patient information provided to answer the questions that follow. Each question or incomplete statement is followed by several suggested answers or completions. Select the one that BEST answers the question or completes the statement. *PRINT THE LETTER OF THE CORRECT ANSWER IN THE SPACE AT THE RIGHT.*

Demographics: 2-year-old male
Chief complaint: Parents complain that the child cannot fixate
Secondary complaint: White reflex in right eye
Medications taken by patient: Nil
Patient's ocular history: Nil
Patient's medical history: Nil
Family ocular history: Nil
Family medical history: Nil
Examination: BCVA – OD-OS - not possible as child is not very young
Pupils: NSNR both eyes
Slit lamp examination: Not done
IOP: 16 mmHg in both eyes
Fundus: OD – Not visible; OS – C:D::0.3:1, foveal reflex is normal

1. What problem can be expected during surgery for cataract extraction with IOL in this child? 1.______
   A. Difficulty in entering the anterior chamber
   B. Collapse of eyeball when the eye is opened
   C. Higher risk of positive vitreous pressure
   D. All of the above

2. Expected complications for this patient include all of the following EXCEPT increased incidence of 2.______
   A. uveitis
   B. after cataract
   C. retinal detachment
   D. vitreous loss

3. The disadvantages of primary capsulotomy include: 3.______
   I. Can cause extension of tear
   II. Can cause IOL dislocation
   III. Can create a situation that it is impossible to place IOL

   A. I and II
   B. II and III
   C. I, II and III
   D. None of the above

4. The disadvantages of secondary posterior capsulotomy can include: 4.______
   I. Can lead to amblyopia
   II. Second surgery required
   III. The cutting of posterior capsule causes dislocation of IOL very frequently

   A. I and II B. II and III C. I and III D. I, II, and III

5. The best method to perform primary capsulotomy is 5.______
   A. Can-opener technique
   B. Posterior continuous curvilinear capsulotomy
   C. Envelope capsulotomy
   D. All of the above

6. The advantages of posterior capsulorrhexis include all EXCEPT 6.______
   A. resists peripheral extension of tear
   B. holds vitreous in place
   C. in-bag implantation of IOL impossible
   D. is an easily mastered technique compared to other forms of capsulotomy

7. The reason why primary anterior vitrectomy is performed is 7.______
   A. anterior vitreous face acts as scaffold for lens epithelial cells
   B. anterior vitreous face acts as scaffold for metaplastic pigment epithelial cells
   C. anterior vitreous face supports exudates and cells that result from break in blood aqueous barrier
   D. all of the above

8. The purpose of anterior vitrectomy while operating congenital cataract is to remove 8.______
   A. entire cortical vitreous
   B. central anterior vitreous
   C. peripheral anterior vitreous
   D. all of the above

9. The posterior continous curvilinear capsulotomy diameter should be 9.______
   A. 1.0 mm to 1.5 mm smaller than the IOL optic
   B. same size as IOL optic
   C. 1.0 mm to 1.5 mm larger than the IOL optic
   D. any of the above

10. The ideal IOL to be used in surgery of paediatric cataract is 10.______
    A. heparin coated one piece IOL with 6 degree angulation of haptic
    B. heparin coated three piece IOL
    C. non-heparin coated one piece IOL
    D. any of the above

11. Which is NOT true of lensectomy with anterior vitrectomy technique? 11.______
    A. Provides clear visual axis
    B. Does not need visual rehabilitation for aphakia by use of spectacles or contact lens
    C. Useful in rubella cataract
    D. Useful in cataract associated with uveitis

12. What is the capsulotomy of choice in paediatric cataracts? 12.______
    A. Anterior curvilinear continous capsulorrhexis with primary posterior continous curvilinear capsulotomy
    B. Can-opener technique
    C. Primary posterior continous curvilinear capsulotomy and anterior can opener technique
    D. Any of the above

13. Which of these treatment strategies is wrong? 13.______
    A. Unilateral cataract should be operated before three months of age
    B. In child less than 2 years, we should use spectacles or contact lenses after lens extraction is done
    C. In child more than 2 years, implant IOL after lens extraction is done
    D. Anterior vitrectomy should not be done if child is less than 2 years

14. Which of the following is NOT true about the silicone contact lenses that are used for correction of paediatric aphakia? 14.______
    A. Have high gas permeability
    B. Cannot correct even minimal astigmatism
    C. Excellent for extended wear purposes
    D. Have high cost

15. Which statement is false? 15.______
    A. If child is less than 2 years, under-correct the refractive error by 20%
    B. If child is between 2 and 8 years, under-correct the refractive error by 10% using IOL
    C. If child is more than 8 years, use IOL to give emmetropia and no under-correction is recommended
    D. None of the above

16. Which IOL is not indicated in children? 16.______
    I. Anterior chamber IOL
    II. Scleral fixated IOL
    III. Posterior chamber IOL

    A. I and II
    B. II and III
    C. I and III
    D. None of the above

17. When should antiamblyopia therapy begin? 17.______
    A. First day after surgery
    B. At first week after surgery
    C. At 10th day after surgery
    D. At one month after surgery

18. What is the most common cause for congenital cataract? 18.______
    A. Chromosomal disorder
    B. Dermatological disorder
    C. Metabolic disorder
    D. Idiopathic

19. What is not true of the pars plana approach for cataract extraction? 19.______
    A. Increased chance of incomplete cataract removal
    B. Increased chance of lens-vitreous mix
    C. This approach is used when no IOL implantation is intended
    D. There is no increased chance of vitreous hemorrhage

20. Which of the following is not a common complication of cataract surgery with IOL implantation in children? 20.______
    A. Retained lens matter
    B. Glaucoma in immediate post-operative period
    C. Cystoid macular edema
    D. Inflammatory reaction

Demographics: 10-year-old female
Chief complaint: Recurrent periorbital swelling right eye from one year
Secondary complaint: Mild drooping of upper lid of right eye
Medications taken by patient: Nil
Patient's ocular history: Nil
Patient's medical history: Nil
Family ocular history: Nil
Family medical history: Nil
Examination: BCVA – OD 6/6; OS 6/6
Pupils: NSNR
Slit lamp examination: Anterior segment is normal
IOP: 20 mmHg in both eyes
Fundus: C:D:: 0.3:1, foveal reflex is normal in both eyes
CT scan: Shows a cystic ring-enhancing lesion with pinhead area of increased attenuation in superior rectus muscle of right eye

21. What is the most appropriate management of this condition? 21.______
    A. Systemic steroids and oral albendazole for 40 days
    B. Systemic steroids only
    C. Oral albendazole only for 40 days
    D. Excision of cyst

22. What is the mode of action of oral albendazole? 22.______
    A. Increased calcium influx
    B. Decreases glucose supply
    C. Causes spastic paralysis of parasite
    D. None of the above

23. Which statement is NOT true for albendazole? 23.______
    A. Take fatty meal to increase bioavailability of albendazole
    B. Steroids decrease albendazole levels
    C. Can treat patients who fail from albendazole treatment with praziquantel
    D. Give injection decadron 4 mg/day for 4 days prior to albendazole

24. Which of the treatment modalities is not correct? 24.______
    A. Treat intraocular cysticerci when live
    B. If subretinal cysticerci is within 8 mm from macula, do subretinal extraction of cyst
    C. If cyst in choroids, incise sclera over it and cyst pops out
    D. For submacular cyst, do vitrectomy and induce retinotomy and then laser barrage

25. What can be the cure of subconjunctival cyst? 25.______
    I. Surgical excision
    II. Spontaneous extrusion
    III. Cure with systemic steroids

    A. I and II B. II and III C. I and III D. I, II and III

26. What is not true for the treatment aspect of an intraocular cyst? 26.______
    A. Though surgical outcome is successful but functional outcome is poor
    B. If intraocular parasite is left untreated it eventually dies after 2-4 years releasing toxins which induces inflammatory reaction
    C. Medical treatment has no role in intraocular cysticerci due to potential sight threatening side effects of toxin release from death of parasite
    D. Systemic steroids is the best treatment option

27. What parasites can cause cystic lesions in the orbit? 27.______
    I. Hydatid cyst II. Cysticercus
    III. Roundworm IV. Tapeworm

    A. I and II B. II and III C. III and IV D. I, II, III, IV

28. Which is not true of the drug praziquantel? 28.______
    A. Praziquantel should be taken with meal rich in carbohydrate
    B. Steroids decrease praziquental levels
    C. Praziquantel causes spastic paralysis of parasite and this is caused by increased calcium influx
    D. All of the above

29. Which is not a feature of cysticercus infection in a patient? 29.______
    A. Rise in eosinophil count
    B. On ultrasound ring shaped lesion with central/marginal echogenic nodule representing scolex
    C. Cysticercus gives starry night appearance on MRI
    D. Anemia

30. What can be the presentation of extraocular muscle involvement? 30.______
    A. Double depressor palsy
    B. Duane's retraction syndrome
    C. Non-specific orbital myositis
    D. All of the above

KEY (CORRECT ANSWERS)

1. D	11. B	21. A
2. C	12. A	22. B
3. C	13. D	23. B
4. A	14. B	24. B
5. B	15. D	25. A
6. D	16. A	26. D
7. D	17. A	27. A
8. B	18. D	28. D
9. A	19. D	29. D
10. A	20. C	30. D

TEST 2

DIRECTIONS: Use the patient information provided to answer the questions that follow. Each question or incomplete statement is followed by several suggested answers or completions. Select the one that BEST answers the question or completes the statement. *PRINT THE LETTER OF THE CORRECT ANSWER IN THE SPACE AT THE RIGHT.*

Demographics: 40-year-old male
Chief complaint: Central black scotoma
Secondary complaint: Nil
Medications taken by patient: Nil
Patient's ocular history: Similar complaints in the past once or twice a year for last three years
Patient's medical history: Patient had pulmonary tuberculosis – treated for 9 months
Family ocular history: Nil
Family medical history: Nil
Examination: BCVA – OD 6/12 improved to 6/6 with +0.5D lens; OS 6/6
Pupils: NSNR
Slit lamp: Anterior segment is normal, serous elevation of retina in posterior segment
IOP: 20 mmHg in both eyes
Fundus: Circumscribed round or oval area of retinal elevation in the macula. The foveal reflex may be absent.
FA: Site of leakage of serous fluid from the RPE into the subretinal space.

1. What are the best management options for this disease? 1.______
   A. Systemic steroids
   B. Argon laser photocoagulation
   C. Wait and watch for four months if it is first episode
   D. Acetazolamide

2. What is not the indication of laser treatment for this disease? 2.______
   A. Bilateral disease
   B. Occupational reason
   C. To increase gain of final visual acuity
   D. If no recovery for 4 months

3. Which of the following is a true feature of laser treatment used for this disease? 3.______
   A. Argon laser is used
   B. Direct laser photocoagulation is effective
   C. Indirect laser photocoagulation is not effective
   D. All of the above

4. Which drug is contraindicated in the management of this patient? 4.______
   A. Steroids
   B. Acetazolamide
   C. Ibuprofen
   D. None of the above

5. What is the most recent mode of laser treatment recommended for this type of patient? 5.______
   A. PDT
   B. TTT
   C. Focal photocoagulation with argon laser
   D. Grid photocoagulation with argon laser

6. What is the role of acetazolamide in this disease? 6.______
   A. Decreases production of aqueous humor
   B. Maintains appropriate kidney function
   C. Enhances resolution of subretinal fluid by promoting RPE pump
   D. All of the above

7. What is not an indication of prompt laser photocoagulation in this disease? 7.______
   A. RPE leak at 1/4 DD away from fovea
   B. Evidence of permanent loss of acuity due to previous episode
   C. Occupational reasons
   D. Detachment present for four months or later

8. What is not a complication following laser photocoagulation? 8.______
   A. Foveal damage
   B. Traction lines
   C. Iatrogenic CNV
   D. Glaucoma

9. Which of the following can resemble this disease in clinical presentation? 9.______
   A. ARMD
   B. Kranenberg's syndrome
   C. Tumors
   D. All of the above

10. What statement is not true regarding CSR? 10.______
   A. The most common location for a leakage point is in the upper nasal quadrant
   B. The lower temporal quadrant is the least likely area to contain a leakage point
   C. All leakage points are within a 1 mm area around the fovea
   D. CSR is a clinical diagnosis and fluorescein angiography is indicated if one decides to laser the lesion

Demographics: 30-year-old male
Chief complaint: Diminution of vision in both eyes – OD > OS
Secondary complaint: Nil
Medications taken by patient: Systemic steroids during previous episodes
Patient's ocular history: Nil
Patient's medical history: Nil
Family ocular history: Not significant
Family medical history: Father had tuberculosis
Examination: BCVA – OD 6/12; OS 6/9
Pupils: NSNR
Slit lamp: Anterior segment is within normal limits
IOP: 16 mm Hg in both eyes
Fundus: Bilateral multiple retinal vein branches occluded in peripheral fundus

11. During follow-up of this patient what are the points to be watched? 11.______

I. Sudden diminution of vision
II. Formation of neovascularisation of disc
III. Formation of neovascularisation elsewhere

A. I and II B. II and III C. I, II and III D. I and III

12. The formation of glial tissue at the posterior pole can have the following sequalae: 12.______

I. Detachment of macula
II. Formation of folds from glial contraction
III. Glial tissue can cover the macula
IV. Rhegmatogenous retinal detachment

A. I, II and III B. II, III and IV C. I, III and IV D. I, II, III, IV

13. Which of the following is not a stage in Eales disease? 13.______

A. Inflammation
B. Ischemia
C. Neovacularisation
D. Proliferation

14. Which of the following is not a treatment modality of Eales disease? 14.______

A. Oral steroids
B. Antitubercular therapy
C. Selective retinal ablation by scatter photocoagulation
D. Antiarthiritic drugs

15. Which of these photocoagulation procedures is useful in treatment of Eales disease? 15.______
    A. Anchoring photocoagulation
    B. PDT
    C. TTT
    D. Focal photocoagulation

16. What cannot be a complication of Eales disease? 16.______
    A. Rubeosis iridis
    B. Hemorrhagic glaucoma
    C. Cataract
    D. Conjunctivitis

17. What is the most frequent cause of visual loss in Eales disease? 17.______
    A. Vitreous hemorrhage
    B. Cataract
    C. Glaucoma
    D. Retinal detachment

18. What is not true about Eales disease? 18.______
    A. Macula is involved early in disease
    B. Most eyes retain good visual acuity
    C. Peripheral scatter photocoagulation of ischemic retina is the treatment of choice for the neovascularisation of Eales disease
    D. Vitrectomy can be employed for removing persistent vitreous hemorrhage and fibrosis

19. What is not true about the non-perfusion in Eales disease? 19.______
    A. Peripheral non-perfusion is present in all patients
    B. The extent of non-perfusion ranges from small areas in far periphery to massive non-perfusion extending into posterior pole
    C. The non-perfusion is usually confluent and sharply demarcated from posterior perfused retina
    D. The nasal retina is most commonly affected by non-perfusion

20. Which of the following can mimic Eales disease? 20.______
    A. Diabetes mellitus
    B. Sickle cell hemoglobinopathy
    C. Sarcoidosis
    D. All of the above

Demographics: 10-year-old male
Chief complaint: Drooping of left upper lid since childhood
Secondary complaint: Nil
Medications taken by patient: Nil
Patient's ocular history: Nil
Patient's medical history: Nil
Family ocular history: Nil
Family medical history: Nil
Examination: BCVA – OD 6/6; OS 6/6
Pupils: OD = OS = NSNR
Slit lamp: Anterior segment is within normal limits in both eyes
IOP: 16 mm Hg in both eyes
Fundus: Both eyes – C:D::0.3:1, foveal reflex is normal
Width of palpebral aperture: Right eye – 10 mm; Left eye – 7 mm
LPS action: Right eye – 11 mm; Left eye – 10 mm

21. This congenital ptosis is 21.______
    A. mild B. moderate C. severe D. none

22. The LPS action in this child is 22.______
    A. good B. fair C. poor D. none

23. What clinical feature can provide a clue for poor LPS action? 23.______
    A. Absence of lid fold
    B. Upper eyelid on eversion as the child looks down does not revert on its own
    C. Child throwing head back
    D. All of the above

24. Which examination is not absolutely essential when the child is to be taken for ptosis surgery? 24.______
    A. Corneal sensation B. Ocular motility
    C. Bell's phenomenon D. Fundus examination

25. Which is the most appropriate treatment measure for this child? 25.______
    A. LPS resection B. Fasanella Servat
    C. Sling surgery D. All of the above

26. What is the most appropriate treatment measure if Marcus Gunn phenomenon is associated with ptosis? 26.______
    A. LPS resection
    B. Fasanella Servat
    C. Sling surgery on the affected side
    D. Sling surgery on both sides

27. Which statement is NOT true of conjunctival approach levator resection? 27.______
    A. It is simple to perform
    B. Recovery period is short
    C. Procedure is not indicated if maximum correction is needed
    D. Should overcorrection occur, treatment is by removing sutures

28. Which statement is true of congenital ptosis? 28.______
    A. Overcorrection is needed
    B. Palpebral aperture width is more in downgaze than in upgaze
    C. It can be associated with Marcus Gunn phenomenon or blepharophimosis syndrome
    D. All of the above

29. The common complications of LPS resection include all of the following EXCEPT 29.______
    A. overcorrection
    B. undercorrection
    C. poor eyelid contour
    D. lid lag

30. All of the following procedures are needed to correct blepharophimosis syndrome EXCEPT 30.______
    A. Verwey's Y-V operation
    B. transnasal fixation
    C. Fasanella Servat
    D. Agnew's lateral canthoplasty

KEY (CORRECT ANSWERS)

1. C	11. C	21. B
2. C	12. D	22. A
3. D	13. D	23. D
4. A	14. D	24. D
5. A	15. A	25. A
6. C	16. D	26. D
7. A	17. A	27. A
8. D	18. A	28. D
9. D	19. D	29. D
10. C	20. D	30. C

TEST 3

DIRECTIONS: Use the patient information provided to answer the questions that follow. Each question or incomplete statement is followed by several suggested answers or completions. Select the one that BEST answers the question or completes the statement. *PRINT THE LETTER OF THE CORRECT ANSWER IN THE SPACE AT THE RIGHT.*

Demographics: 10-year-old male
Chief complaint: Drooping of left upper lid since childhood
Secondary complaint: Nil
Medications taken by patient: Nil
Patient's ocular history: Nil
Patient's medical history: Nil
Family ocular history: Nil
Family medical history: Nil
Examination: BCVA – OD 6/6; OS 6/6
Pupils: OD = OS = NSNR
Slit lamp: Anterior segment is within normal limits in both eyes
IOP: 16 mm Hg in both eyes
Fundus: Both eyes – C:D::0.3:1, foveal reflex is normal
Width of palpebral aperture: Right eye – 10 mm; Left eye – 7 mm
LPS action: Right eye – 11 mm; Left eye – 10 mm

1. All of the following can cause an impression of pseudoptosis EXCEPT 1.______
   A. hypothalmos B. enophthalmos
   C. epicanthal fold D. distichiatic cilia

2. What is the earliest time that surgery should be performed for congenital ptosis? 2.______
   A. Immediately at birth
   B. At 3-4 years of age
   C. At 10 years of age
   D. At 15 years of age

3. Which of the following can be employed to diagnose myasthenia gravis associated ptosis? 3.______
   A. Electromyography
   B. Serum assay for cholinergic receptor antibodies
   C. Chest x-ray
   D. All of the above

4. Which treatment measure is NOT appropriate for a patient of myasthenia gravis? 4.______
   A. Regular physical exercises B. Immunosuppressives
   C. Plasmapheresis D. Oral neostigmine

5. Which of the following is true regarding autogenous fascia lata sling surgery? 5.______
   A. It cannot be done in children younger than three years of age
   B. Even in unilateral sever ptosis, a bilateral fascia lata sling surgery is performed
   C. For obtaining fascia lata strip, an incision is given on the line joining the head of fibula and anterior superior iliac spine
   D. All of the above

6. Which of the following is NOT true of the congenital ptosis associated with superior rectus weakness? 6.______
   A. The superior rectus weakness associated with congenital ptosis is myogenic
   B. The hypertropia has to be corrected before doing any ptosis surgery
   C. The needed levator resection in this patient is less than that required if superior rectus weakness is not associated with ptosis
   D. Superior rectus weakness is associated with congenital ptosis as the two muscles develop from the same myotome

7. The indications of brow suspension include all of the following EXCEPT 7.______
   A. unilateral severe ptosis
   B. failed ptosis surgery
   C. mild ptosis
   D. misdirected third nerve palsy

8. Which of the following is a prerequisite for brow suspension? 8.______
   A. Good Bell's phenomenon
   B. Normal corneal sensation
   C. Normal ocular movements
   D. All of the above

Demographics: 50-year-old male
Chief complaint: Heaviness and pain in both eyes from three years
Secondary complaint: Headache off and on
Medications taken by patient: Timolol 0.5% eye drops, twice a day
Patient's ocular history: Uses glasses with power of +2.0 Dsph
Patient's medical history: Nil
Family ocular history: Father had blinding disease of eye
Family medical history: Nil
Examination: BCVA – OD 6/12; OS 6/12
Pupils: OD = OS = NSNR
Slit lamp: Anterior segment is within normal limits in both eyes; early cataract in both eyes
IOP: 20 mmHg in both eyes
Fundus: OD – C:D::0.6:1, foveal reflex is normal; OS – C:D::0.7:1, foveal reflex is normal

9. What can be the probable cause of diminution of vision in this patient? 9.______
   A. Glaucoma
   B. Cataract
   C. ARMD
   D. All of the above

10. What is not true about topical timolol used in control of IOP in open-angle glaucoma patients? 10.______
    A. It is non-selective β-blocker
    B. It does not cause bronchoconstriction
    C. It does not have any intrinsic sympathomimetic activity
    D. It has a measurable ocular hypotensive effect

11. Which is true of topical betaxolol? 11.______
    A. It is a cardioselective β-1 adrenergic blocker
    B. The IOP reduction with betaxolol is less than that seen with timolol
    C. The visual field is preserved better with betaxolol than timolol
    D. All of the above

12. The systemic carbonic anhydrase inhibitor that can be used to lower IOP is 12.______
    A. methazolamide
    B. ethoxzolamide
    C. dichlorphenamide
    D. all of the above

13. Which is not true of the topical carbonic anhydrase inhibitors that can lower IOP? 13.______
    A. Sezolamide and dorzolamide are drugs in this group
    B. MK 927 is also a drug of this group
    C. 1% dorzolamide is used topically in patients with glaucoma
    D. Ocular side effects include stinging and burning

14. Which is not true of apraclonidine hydrochloride? 14.______
    A. It is a selective α-2 agonist
    B. It decreases IOP by β-blocker mechanism
    C. It reduces the incidence of IOP spies after anterior segment laser procedures such as YAG capsulotomy
    D. The common systemic side effects are sensation of dry mouth and nose

15. The mechanism of action if brimonidine in patients with open-angle glaucoma does NOT include 15.______
    A. reduction of aqueous humor production
    B. increased uveo-scleral outflow
    C. neuroprotective role as it causes upregulation of the receptors of neuronal factors
    D. causes pupil constriction

16. Which of the following is not true of latanoprost? 16.______
    A. It is a PGF_2 alpha agonist
    B. It should be instilled early in the morning
    C. It is used in concentration of 0.005% once a day
    D. It causes an increase in uveo-scleral outflow

17. The ocular side effects of pilocarpine include 17.______
    A. spasm of accommodation
    B. conjunctival hyperemia
    C. myopia
    D. all of the above

18. Which of the following is NOT true about topical dorzolamide? 18.______
    A. It has poor corneal penetration
    B. It is additive to pilocarpine and timolol in lowering IOP
    C. The most frequent side effect is bitter taste
    D. It can be used in patients with cardiovascular and pulmonary disease

19. Which of the following is true of topical latanoprost? 19.______
    A. It reduces IOP without reducing aqueous production
    B. It is additive to all aqueous humor suppressants known
    C. It does not lose efficacy over time
    D. All of the above

20. Which of the following agents can be used in neuroprotection in glaucoma? 20.______
    A. Calcium channel blockers
    B. Brimonidine
    C. NMDA antagonist
    D. All of the above

21. What laser procedure is specifically indicated in treatment of patients with open-angle glaucoma? 21.______
    A. YAG laser peripheral iridectomy
    B. Argon laser peripheral iridectomy
    C. Argon laser trabeculoplasty
    D. Laser pupilloplasty

22. The systemic side effects of topical pilocarpine include 22.______
    A. Diaphoresis
    B. Stimulation of glands including salivary and lacrimal
    C. Increased bronchial secretion
    D. All of the above

23. Which of the following is NOT true about retinal detachment that results from the use of topical pilocarpine? 23.______
    A. The retinal detachment is of inflammatory origin
    B. These are typically rhegmatogenous retinal detachments
    C. It is presumed that ciliary body contraction exerts vitreo-retinal traction that causes retinal tears
    D. The degree of risk appears to be related to the pre-existing retinal pathology

24. The ocular side effects of topical epinephrine do NOT include 24.______
    A. allergic blepharoconjunctivitis
    B. adrenochrome deposits
    C. madarosis
    D. headache

25. Which is NOT a feature of dipivefrin? 25.______
    A. It is significantly more lipophilic than epinephrine
    B. It has better corneal penetration than epinephrine
    C. The compound is hydrolyzed to epinephrine after absorption into the eye with majority of hydrolysis occurring in the cornea
    D. None of the above

26. The intraocular side effects of epinephrine do NOT include 26.______
    A. mydriasis
    B. madarosis
    C. corneal endothelial damage
    D. epinephrine maculopathy

27. The systemic side effects of oral carbonic anhydrase inhibitors include all of the following EXCEPT 27.______
    A. metabolic alkalosis
    B. paresthesias
    C. hypokalemia
    D. renal calculi

28. Which statement is not true of intravenous mannitol used in control of IOP? 28.______
    A. A dose of 2 g/kg body weight of a 20% solution is to be given intravenously in 30 minutes
    B. The onset of action is 20-60 minutes and the duration varies from two to six hours
    C. It is less efficacious than oral glycerol
    D. It is rapidly excreted unmetabolized in urine

29. The indications of trabeculectomy in a patient of open-angle glaucoma include all of the following EXCEPT: 29.______
    A. A patient whose IOP is not controlled even with use of two topical anti-glaucoma medications
    B. A patient with failed argon laser trabeculoplasty
    C. Angle closure glaucoma but with no peripheral anterior synechiae
    D. A patient who has advanced open-angle glaucoma but is expected to be poor with follow up

30. The complications of laser procedure for treatment of glaucoma include 30.______
    A. an immediate rise in IOP
    B. iritis
    C. formation of peripheral anterior synechiae in laser trabeculoplasty
    D. all of the above

KEY (CORRECT ANSWERS)

1. D	11. D	21. C
2. B	12. D	22. D
3. D	13. C	23. A
4. A	14. B	24. D
5. D	15. D	25. D
6. C	16. B	26. B
7. C	17. D	27. A
8. D	18. A	28. C
9. D	19. D	29. C
10. B	20. D	30. D

www.ingramcontent.com/pod-product-compliance
Lightning Source LLC
LaVergne TN
LVHW081639021025
822565LV00018B/1667